# THE MEDICAL SCIENCE OF HOUSE, M.D.

# The Medical Science of
# House, M.D.

## Andrew Holtz

BERKLEY BOULEVARD, NEW YORK

**The Berkley Publishing Group**
**Published by the Penguin Group**
**Penguin Group (USA) Inc.**
**375 Hudson Street, New York, New York 10014, USA**
Penguin Group (Canada), 90 Eglinton Avenue East, Suite 700, Toronto, Ontario M4P 2Y3, Canada
(a division of Pearson Penguin Canada Inc.)
Penguin Books Ltd., 80 Strand, London WC2R 0RL, England
Penguin Group Ireland, 25 St. Stephen's Green, Dublin 2, Ireland (a division of Penguin Books Ltd.)
Penguin Group (Australia), 250 Camberwell Road, Camberwell, Victoria 3124, Australia
(a division of Pearson Australia Group Pty. Ltd.)
Penguin Books India Pvt. Ltd., 11 Community Centre, Panchsheel Park, New Delhi—110 017, India
Penguin Group (NZ), Cnr. Airborne and Rosedale Roads, Albany, Auckland 1310, New Zealand
(a division of Pearson New Zealand Ltd.)
Penguin Books (South Africa) (Pty.) Ltd., 24 Sturdee Avenue, Rosebank, Johannesburg 2196,
South Africa

Penguin Books Ltd., Registered Offices: 80 Strand, London WC2R 0RL, England

While the author has made every effort to provide accurate telephone numbers and Internet addresses at
the time of publication, neither the publisher nor the author assumes any responsibility for errors, or for
changes that occur after publication. Further, publisher does not have any control over and does not assume any responsibility for author or third-party websites or their content.

This book was not authorized, prepared, approved, licensed, or endorsed by any entity involved in creating or producing the *House, M.D.* television series.

PRINTING HISTORY
Berkley Boulevard trade paperback edition / October 2006

Library of Congress Cataloging-in-Publication Data

Holtz, Andrew.
   The medical science of House, M.D. / Andrew Holtz.
      p. cm.
   ISBN 0-425-21230-0
   1. Medicine—Miscellanea.   2. Medical care—Miscellanea.   3. Medicine on television.
   4. House, M.D.   I. Title

   R702.H63 2006
   610—dc22                                                          2006042989

PRINTED IN THE UNITED STATES OF AMERICA

10  9  8  7  6  5  4  3  2  1

To my parents, Merriman and Carolyn Holtz,
for their love and support, which has given me astonishing opportunities.

To my wife, Kelly Butler Holtz,
for her love and companionship;
but particularly for managing our home and
family while this book was being written.

To our children, Aaron and Judy,
for putting up with my absences for long workdays.

# CONTENTS

**Introduction: Tracking Zebras** . . . . . . . . . . . . . . . . . . . ix

**1. "Doc, I Don't Feel So Good"** . . . . . . . . . . . . . . . . . . . . 1

The presentation of patients to physicians. Most complaints are common, but every now and then there is a "zebra" lurking in the exam room.

**2. Poking and Probing** . . . . . . . . . . . . . . . . . . . . . . . . 28

The exam. The clues physicians look for.

**3. Let's Run Some Tests** . . . . . . . . . . . . . . . . . . . . . . . 54

The tests and devices used to peer inside patients.

**4. Is There a Computer in the House?** . . . . . . . . . . . . . . 86

There is just too much information for any physician to know everything and too little time to manually sort through all the data produced by labs and scanners.

**5. The Whiteboard** . . . . . . . . . . . . . . . . . . . . . . . . . . 101

Twins of House's precious whiteboard are in every hospital, full of scribbles listing patient symptoms, likely and unlikely causes, and possible alternatives.

# CONTENTS

**6. Let's Make You Better** . . . . . . . . . . . . . . . . . . . . . . . **126**

Choosing the right treatment to fit the disease. A complete cure may be elusive and the options aren't always ideal.


**7. Bedside Manner** . . . . . . . . . . . . . . . . . . . . . . . . . . . . **169**

House tries to avoid patients, but understanding the patient as a whole person, not just a list of symptoms, is central to complete medical care. House's reliance on powerful painkillers raises questions . . . as does his sense of ethics.


**8. No Doctor Is an Island** . . . . . . . . . . . . . . . . . . . . . . . **212**

Physicians are just one part of teams of health care professionals. Hospitals are communities with hierarchies and cultures, governed by rules and regulations, and monitored by professional groups and government.


**Epilogue** . . . . . . . . . . . . . . . . . . . . . . . . . . . . . . . . . . **245**

**Index** . . . . . . . . . . . . . . . . . . . . . . . . . . . . . . . . . . . . . **247**

# Tracking Zebras

Every medical student hears this wisdom about diagnosis: "When you hear hoofbeats behind you, don't expect to see a zebra." Outside of Africa, of course, hoofbeats usually signal a horse.

*House, M.D.* features a team of medical specialists, led by Dr. Gregory House, that is in the business of tracking medical zebras, those astonishing cases where hoofbeats do not announce horses at all. When a young, apparently healthy woman suddenly has a seizure and loses her ability to speak, House and his team find a tapeworm in her brain, not the tumor that was first suspected. When a sixteen-year-old rugby player has double vision, the cause is not a collision on the playing field, it is a mutated virus lodged in his brain.

The character of Gregory House is partly based on the famous fictional detective Sherlock Holmes, and like Holmes, Dr. House is ready to grab hold of unlikely solutions to the mysteries confronting him, once all the other possibilities have been ruled out. Admittedly, the physicians on *House, M.D.* see a skewed case mix, and the diseases they uncover are frequently beyond one-in-a-million rarities, but that fact does not mean the cases are impossibly fanciful. If you distill the experience of thousands of physicians and millions of patients over many years, well, anything that can happen probably has. Tapeworms and mutant viruses are indeed found, albeit rarely, in the brains of real patients by physicians who had no idea that a medical zebra would knock on their doors that particular day.

And while Gregory House performs his feats of diagnosis with more speed, flair, and bravado than workaday doctors, he does what all physicians try to do when faced with a puzzling case: He makes critical connections between faint clues in order to identify and treat, in time, the medical perils threatening his patients.

So how do physicians, at a local medical office, hospital emergency department, or major academic medical center, determine whether the complaints of their patients are routine or startling? In the pages ahead, we will tour the methods and tools of medical diagnosis and treatment, in order to understand the fact and fiction of *House, M.D.*

Every case is full of unknowns at first . . . and every physician must quickly make preliminary judgments from fragments of information. Is the problem immediately life-threatening? Is it contagious? Is intervention needed now, or is there time to investigate all the possibilities? Is talking to the patient and performing a quick physical examination sufficient, or are lab tests, scans, or other special procedures called for?

Physicians ask questions. They do a top-to-bottom inventory of their patients' organ systems. They may order tests, scans, or diagnostic procedures that will help them rule in or out different possible diagnoses. Many of the questions and choices along the diagnostic decision-tree are affected by the setting of the doctor-patient encounter. A family physician may be able to link new symptoms with a chronic condition the patient has been dealing with for years. An emergency physician will act to rapidly determine whether the patient's life or limbs are in immediate peril. A specialist will seek to answer the specific questions that brought the patient to his or her practice. An oncologist will look for a tumor. An infectious disease specialist will look for an infection. A pulmonologist will inspect the lungs. And so on.

While the basic diagnostic methodology applied by physicians today has been in use for a century or more, the technological tools now available allow physicians to quickly see things that their predecessors often could observe only too late, during an autopsy. Electron microscopes, monoclonal antibody tests, ultrasound, CT scans and MRI imaging, and many more devices and techniques can be brought to bear. But these tools do not make the diagnosis; physicians decide when and how to apply specific tests, and then how to interpret the results.

Here then is a journey toward diagnosis.

# ONE

# "Doc, I Don't Feel So Good"

A twenty-nine-year-old female who suffered a seizure and lost the ability to speak. A man with a heart rate so fast it couldn't pump blood effectively. A fifteen-year-old model who suddenly became violently aggressive and then passed out.

These are some of House's mysteries.

At first, every patient is a mystery. Many are solved in moments. Others take longer. And some are never solved. Gregory House, M.D., and his team on *House, M.D.* tackle tough, even bizarre, cases in each episode; but almost every patient comes to them with a medical history, even if vital questions are unanswered. Each patient has seen several physicians and had a series of tests. House knows that the patient has a serious problem, and one that isn't explained by the usual suspects.

By the time a woman who is sleeping eighteen hours a day comes to the attention of Dr. House in "Fidelity" (1-07), she's already been seen by three emergency department physicians, two neurologists, and a radiologist; so the obvious diagnosis, depression, has already been considered and discarded. And when a fresh college grad is spasming with shocklike sensations, other physicians have already investigated vitamin deficiency, cancers, multiple sclerosis, neuropathies, and some toxic exposures before handing off the patient to Dr. House's team.

Symptoms are, of course, critical bits of information needed to make a proper diagnosis. But one set of symptoms often can point to several diseases. This list of options is known as the "differential diagnosis." A sudden fever, sore throat, and muscle weakness are symptoms of the flu. But the same set of symptoms is also caused by dengue fever and a variety of other viral and bacterial infections. Flulike symptoms are frequently the first sign of HIV infection. Symptoms in isolation can be very difficult to read.

So how do physicians start down the best path toward diagnosis?

Context is everything. For example, when a patient has recently traveled to the tropics, then dengue fever moves higher up the list. But before a physician gets to the patient's medical and personal history, before the patient and physician have exchanged a single word, a key piece of information is known: the setting in which the patient first presents himself.

In medical parlance, "to present" is to come before a medical professional with a problem or complaint. Presentation is the initial circumstance of the patient-provider interaction, before there is any examination, before any tests are done. The patient either feels something is wrong or something happens, a collapse or seizure, which prompts someone to bring the patient in for medical attention.

The initial circumstances largely determine the initial diagnostic process. Did the patient arrive by ambulance? Did she walk into an after-hours clinic? Did he make an appointment in advance to see his regular primary care physician? Dr. House looks at his clinic patients much differently than he does the challenging cases that are referred

2

to him. He assumes clinic patients have common maladies. Indeed, in "Sports Medicine" (1-12), he diagnoses four patients in less than three minutes, all in the clinic waiting area. On the other hand, Dr. House regularly strikes out the common diagnoses on his conference room whiteboard, as he digs deeper to find the rare explanations. The context of the first encounter is a powerful clue.

## Primary Care

"If you are House and you're in that tertiary care center and the patient is in the intensive care unit, the context is that the person is either very sick or has something extremely weird, because they've already made it to that environment," says Rick Kellerman, M.D., who is a family physician in Wichita, Kansas, and the 2006–2007 president of the American Academy of Family Physicians.

"One of the really difficult areas of primary care is that we see people who just walk in off the street. So some people with sore throat are going to have tonsillitis. Once in a while they are going to have cancer of the esophagus."

In many ways, the first doctor to see a patient has the toughest job. For the first doctor, a new patient may be a blank slate. Is the problem life threatening or merely annoying? Will the patient get better on his own, or should the condition be treated?

"I think it is incredibly difficult to diagnose somebody. I think to the public it often looks like it is very easy to do, but it is really quite difficult. Patients don't come in with their diagnosis stamped on their forehead," Dr. Kellerman says.

Patients come in off the street, unselected, with what is called an undifferentiated problem. Perhaps the complaint is tiredness. The challenge is to go from "tiredness" to what is actually going on inside that particular patient.

## "What Brings You in Today?"

An open-ended question like that often begins a typical doctor-patient encounter. But the process of diagnosis often is already under way. The physician may see the patient in the hall or waiting room. Is he sitting upright or bent in pain? Does she appear to be alert or drowsy? Does he walk into the exam room easily or not?

In "Paternity" (1-02), Dr. House looks out from his office at a young patient in the hallway and becomes intrigued by the twitching of one of the boy's legs. The boy and his parents had not paid attention to the muscle spasm, but it turns out to be a critical clue to the cause of the other odd symptoms that brought the boy to the hospital.

---

### Interruptions

Even as physicians ask probing questions of patients, Gregory House is far from the only doctor who interrupts patients' replies.

Two decades ago, researchers recorded dozens of office visits to study the interactions between physicians and patients. On average, the physicians interrupted patients after only eighteen seconds. Less than a quarter of patients were allowed to finish their opening statements about their medical concerns before being cut off.

Over the years, it doesn't look like the situation has improved much. In 1999, other researchers performed an analysis of more than 250 patient visits at the offices of twenty-nine family practice physicians, some of whom had received special training in communication skills. Although the physicians asked patients about their concerns three-quarters of the time, they let those patients finish their answers just over a third of the time. The average time until the first interruption: just twenty-three seconds.

Of course, physicians are pressed for time, but they don't save much by interrupting patients. It took less than thirty seconds on average for patients to finish explaining what they were concerned about.

---

The process that starts with a broad question quickly moves to specifics. If the patient is complaining about a "stomachache," then the doctor asks where exactly the pain is. She may ask the patient to point to the source of the pain. Is it in the area of the stomach? Higher in the esophagus or chest? Down around the intestines or appendix? Is the pain constant or does it come and go and how often? What makes it worse or better? Has the patient vomited?

Stomach pain by itself, like most symptoms in isolation, could mean almost anything. The key to understanding the complaint is to quickly survey the patient's daily life, looking for combinations of circumstances that might narrow the list of possibilities. So the physicians may ask about allergies, hospitalizations, surgeries, chronic illnesses, smoking, alcohol use.

It is also important to know the patient's family situation: married, single, divorced? Any kids? How's work going?

It may seem like stretching things to ask a patient with a stomachache about how things are at home, including perhaps a sexual history, but stress is often linked to abdominal pain and the sexual relationship between spouses may be an indication of stress. More specifically, in women, abdominal pain may be a symptom of pelvic inflammatory disease, perhaps related to sexual history or the use of an intrauterine device (IUD) for contraception. As this example of the various trails leading from a stomachache complaint shows, the initial conversation between physician and patient is actually a sophisticated dance.

Of course, many of the questions lead to dead ends. That's not a bad outcome. Striking things off the list of potential ailments is progress.

Dr. Kellerman likens the initial assessment of a patient to a game of Concentration. Many puzzle pieces are revealed and then turned over again, because they don't match. But with each move the number of squares that might be hiding the piece you are seeking is reduced. The underlying pattern is revealed bit by bit and the goal comes closer step by step.

## Seizures

Seizures strike many of House's patients. Indeed, in the first season almost half the episodes featured a seizure . . . quickly followed by shouts of "Ativan! Stat!"

That rate of seizures seems remarkable, but it may well be within reason for the type of patients seen by House. The sort of seizures usually depicted on the show are sudden bursts of electrical activity in the brain. These brain storms, called epileptic seizures, can have many causes.

"The number of disorders that can give rise to epileptic events is lengthy," says William J. Nowack, M.D., associate professor with the Comprehensive Epilepsy Center at University of Kansas Medical Center in Kansas City.

But having one epileptic seizure does not necessarily mean a person has epilepsy.

"Epilepsy is more than one epileptic seizure or, according to the latest definition, at least one epileptic seizure and a brain lesion that makes other seizures likely. It is a chronic disease. Not every epileptic seizure is a sign of epilepsy. There can be acute things, like an infection of the brain, a tumor, stroke, a head injury, and so on, that irritates the neurons to produce a seizure which occurs close in time to the cause, but the cause comes and then is gone and the seizure does not recur. That's called an acute symptomatic seizure. It doesn't necessarily predict or result in the chronic disease of epilepsy," says Dr. Nowack.

## "Doc, I Don't Feel So Good"

There are also many sudden events that may look like an epileptic seizure but are not, because they don't feature the electrical overload in the patient's brain. Other brain diseases, for instance, can cause movements, jerking, or posturing that can be mistaken for an epileptic seizure. Chronic pain and hyperventilation, irregular heartbeats, or cardiac arrest are some of the many other possible causes of sudden attacks. Some things, like a head injury, may cause epileptic seizures or nonepileptic attacks.

These other things can be just as traumatic as an epileptic seizure, but because they have different causes, they require different responses.

The most frequent response by House's team to an epileptic seizure is a quick injection of Ativan. The generic name of the drug is lorazepam. Taken orally as a tablet or liquid, it can relieve anxiety. Injections of Ativan are commonly used to interrupt seizures. Ativan usually works, but sometimes other medicines are necessary.

"It basically works on the excitability of nerve cells. It makes them less excitable. It does work. If someone is having an epileptic seizure, that's the way you can terminate it and avoid what's called status epilepticus, which is a continuous epileptic event," Dr. Nowack says. "Ativan is not a long-term treatment, but acutely, it's very good."

An Ativan injection must be done carefully, because if the drug goes directly into an artery, it can cause the blood vessel to spasm and shut off blood flow in the area. In severe cases, the result of injecting Ativan into an artery can be gangrene that may require amputation. The drug can also cause excessive sedation.

"Status epilepticus is a medical emergency and the longer it goes on, the higher the complication rate. Since epileptic seizures tend to recur and Ativan is an effective antiseizure treatment for only a limited time, long-term treatment with other medicines also needs to be considered. The treatment team needs to decide whether it is an epileptic

7

event or something else that is being treated, because the team might miss treating the real cause of the problem," Dr. Nowack cautions.

Epileptic seizures of the sort so often seen on *House, M.D.* look frightening. With the patient suddenly convulsing, eyes rolling up, and perhaps choking, it seems obvious that instant action is needed to stop the attack.

"It is a dramatic event, no doubt about it." But Dr. Nowack says that what physicians do after resorting to Ativan is also critical.

"The important thing, after the physicians get the seizure stopped, is to figure out what caused it," he says. "Usually an epileptic seizure by itself lasts less than about two and a half minutes; and that, by itself, probably doesn't cause damage. But they are afraid of going into status epilepticus, repeated, prolonged seizures without a return to consciousness. It can go on for five minutes, ten minutes, half an hour or even longer. And the longer it lasts, the greater is the risk of injury or death.

"It's not an unreasonable approach, the first time a convulsion occurs, to try and stop it and then to sort out what's causing it."

---

If the physician and patient already have a relationship, the diagnostic process can move along quickly. Perhaps the new complaint is another episode of a long-term health issue. When the doctor and patient know each other, the physician will already have a sense of how accurately and fully the patient reports symptoms. Does she minimize pain? Does he exaggerate fatigue? Previous treatments are in the record. So are notations on medications, alcohol, smoking, type and place of work, home environment, and more.

Dr. House often proclaims that, "Everybody lies."

"I don't know if everybody lies intentionally, I don't know if I'd agree with that; but there are certain patients that either through their body language, the way they say things, or the things they say, make your 'suspicion meter' go up. We see this very commonly with alcoholics and drug abusers. Others may not give us the entire sexual history," Dr. Kellerman says. "So there are always things where you have to wonder if you are getting the whole truth."

Despite Dr. House's brash skepticism, most physicians rely on the veracity of what their patients tell them.

"Most people, I figure, if they are in the office, it's because they do have some sort of a problem, there is some suffering that they've got. I try to take them at face value, but you get that gut feeling sometimes that something's just not right," Dr. Kellerman says.

---

## Lying Without Speaking

Dr. House eventually uncovered a lie that helped solve the case in "Failure to Communicate" (2-10) even though the patient did not speak a falsehood . . . at least not the way you might expect.

The patient came to the team's attention after he suddenly began spouting nonsense sentences; a condition called aphasia. The word is from Greek, meaning "without speech." The patient did not understand that the words he used did not make sense to anyone else, because something was wrong with the way his brain was processing language.

"With this type of aphasia the patients seem to think like they speak, that is, they are unaware of the problem and comprehend neither the speech of others nor the problems with their own speech. These patients are often assumed to have a psychosis rather than a neurological disorder since they look okay, walk, eat, and have no physically obvious problem," says James Kelly, M.D., from the University of Colorado School of Medicine in Denver.

In the episode of *House, M.D.*, the clues, like the patient's speech, did not make sense, until Dr. House figured out that the patient had made a trip to South America for experimental brain surgery. He had not told anyone, including his wife. After the secret was uncovered, the problem was determined to be cerebral malaria. That parasitic infection had not been on the list of possibilities because no one knew the patient had traveled to an area where malaria is endemic.

Dr. Kelly, who is a Fellow of the American Academy of Neurology, says that although he has never treated a case of aphasia caused by malaria, there are a few case reports in the medical literature.

Malaria attacks the brain in less than 1 percent of cases, according to the medical textbook *Neurology and General Medicine*. However, when it does happen, the prognosis is often poor. The textbook says up to half of patients with cerebral malaria die.

The choice of treatments depends on the species of parasite and whether the patient was infected in an area where the parasites might be resistant to certain drugs.

---

As with so many aspects of medicine, the skill is not merely reading biological signs and symptoms, it is in understanding the patient as a person. The physician does not merely tote up the symptoms, he or she must weigh the information, judging its accuracy, suspecting what might be missing, and deciding its relevance to the immediate needs of the patient.

---

## Munchausen Syndrome

Karl Friedrich von Münchhausen was an eighteenth-century German nobleman known for telling tall tales. It was said he bragged of riding cannonballs and journeying to the moon. He is credited with the phrase "to pull oneself up by the bootstraps." That is how he claimed to have lifted himself out of the mire in a swamp. Münchhausen's stories were retold and then published by others. His name became synonymous with exaggerations and eventually gained a medical meaning, Munchausen syndrome, which is a psychiatric disorder. Also known generically as factitious illnesses, Munchausen's describes the behavior of people who fabricate medical symptoms, or even injure themselves, in order to receive treatment.

Munchausen's is not the same as malingering. Malingerers have something to gain by pretending to be sick. The classic example is a soldier who feigns illness in order to avoid being sent into combat.

A patient suspected of having Munchausen syndrome was featured in the episode "Deception" (2-09). That episode illustrated one of the greatest risks of the syndrome: that the tests and treatments prescribed on the basis of false information may lead to real harm. The patient underwent a number of invasive procedures, including almost having her bone marrow destroyed by radiation.

Patients may also do real harm to themselves in order to create realistic symptoms. In one case, a person tried to simulate the lung damage of cystic fibrosis. After the patient's death, examination of the lungs found large amounts of crystalline material. Apparently, the patient had breathed in talc. The breathing impairment was quite real, even if the underlying cause was psychiatric and not genetic.

Sometimes the falsehoods and reality intersect. Doctors in England reported the case of a man who claimed he had been diagnosed as HIV positive two years earlier. However, his new blood tests were negative for HIV. Further testing with more sensitive tests discovered that he had recently been infected with HIV. Although he had not been truthful about his earlier test results, in the end he did indeed have an HIV infection.

So even if the patient isn't telling the truth, that does not always mean he or she doesn't really have the disease.

Children are the victims in a disturbing variation of the syndrome called Munchausen by proxy. In this case, the person with the abnormal need for attention is the parent. The psychiatric disturbance causes the parent to harm the child. The parent then gets the attention and sympathy naturally offered to the parent of a sick child.

These cases can be difficult to discover. Sometimes hidden cameras are used when health care professionals suspect that the source of the child's physical symptoms is child abuse by a mentally ill parent or guardian.

Sometimes people with Munchausen syndrome are hidden within the ranks of health care providers. Within the logic of the syndrome, the strong attraction to the health care system can make health care jobs appealing. One of the most notorious cases is that of British nurse Beverly Allitt, who was convicted in 1993 of murdering four children and injecting more than a dozen other young patients with potassium or insulin.

---

When people go to the doctor, they want to know what's wrong. Is it a virus? Could it be cancer? And while sometimes patients tell their physicians what they believe might be causing their complaints, declaring, "I have an infection," or "I've got a tumor," all they really know when they first arrive at the clinic or hospital is that something's not right. We seek care because we hurt or we are tired or constipated or congested. It's the job of the physician to take the complaints presented by patients and then start the search for the cause. Many of the presenting problems fit into a few major categories.

# Common Presenting Problems
# in Primary Care[1]

## WEIGHT LOSS

How much has the patient's weight dropped? If a 200-pound man lost ten pounds in six months without dieting, it could be cause for concern. Everything from depression to cancer to HIV might be considered; although in many cases the cause is never identified.

## FATIGUE

Is it acute or chronic? Acute fatigue could be anything from just not getting enough sleep to problems with medications. Fatigue lasting more than six months is considered chronic. However, fewer than 5 percent of patients meet the official criteria of chronic fatigue syndrome.

## DIZZINESS

Where does the dizziness seem to affect the patient? In the head or the body? One of the first steps is to pin down the type of dizziness. It could be vertigo, which is a sense that things are moving or tilting. Dizziness can be prelude to fainting. It can be felt as a balance problem or unsteadiness when standing or walking. There are also other types of dizziness and it can come and go or last for long periods.

## COUGH

A cough is considered chronic if it lasts more than three weeks. Varieties include postnasal drip, asthma-like symptoms, cough related to heartburn or related problems or other causes.

1. These common presenting problems are highlighted in the *Manual of Family Practice*, Robert B. Taylor, M.D., ed., 2002.

## CHEST PAIN

Is it sudden and sharp enough that the patient couldn't wait for a regular appointment during office hours? That type of symptom is termed emergent chest pain. Chest pain is usually muscle strain, heartburn, or some other relatively minor problem; but it could also be a sign of a heart attack. The physician must quickly determine whether the problem is minor or possibly life threatening. Because time is of the essence when treating a heart attack, the public is usually advised not to wait for a regular appointment, but to seek emergency care, just in case.

## ABDOMINAL PAIN

As with chest pain, the first task is to decide whether the problem is potentially life threatening. Is it an upset stomach or appendicitis?

Other common issues that people bring to primary care physicians include jaundice (a yellow tint to the skin or eyes), swelling, and pain in the pelvic region. Back pain is one of the leading complaints; almost everyone has it at some time or another. It almost always gets better on its own, but chronic back pain is one of the most contentious and frustrating issues facing modern medicine. Back pain can prevent people from working or enjoying other activities, but there are no surefire, simple treatments.

---

### Sexsomnia

Can you have sex in your sleep? That was the explanation that House gave a clinic patient in the episode "Role Model" (1-17). The woman had symptoms of a recent miscarriage, but she denied having had sex in almost a year.

## "Doc, I Don't Feel So Good"

Having sex while sleeping is certainly one step beyond sleepwalking, but at least some experts say it is similar to other behaviors that are called parasomnias. Most people experience parasomnias and other sleep disorders at one time or another. More common parasomnias include bedwetting, night terrors, and even violent attacks that the attacker has no conscious memory of. The causes are not always clear. Sometimes there is an emotional trigger or a traumatic experience that affects sleep. Alcohol and other drugs, including medicines, can affect sleep. But many episodes of various parasomnias may come and go without an easy explanation.

In the fall of 2005, a man in Toronto, Canada, was acquitted of sexual assault because the judge accepted the explanation that he was asleep during the incident. Sleep expert Dr. Colin Shapiro, from the University of Toronto, testified for the defense. He and his colleagues have proposed that sexsomnia should be recognized as a parasomnia.

There are only a few reports of sexsomnia in the medical literature and no one knows how common it may be. The condition can affect both men and women. Some cases, like the one in Toronto, come to light because of a sexual assault complaint. However, in one case, the partner said the patient was actually a more gentle and amorous lover when he was asleep.

Some sexsomnia patients have been treated with clonazepam, which is generally used to treat seizures or anxiety.

Researchers say sexsomnia is not the same as common sexual arousal during sleep.

By the way, the sleeping and eating behavior epitomized by the comic strip character Dagwood also has a basis in fact. For decades, Dagwood has made midnight raids on his refrigerator to down his signature gargantuan sandwiches.

Nocturnal eating (drinking) syndrome is listed in the International

Classification of Sleep Disorders. The syndrome may affect up to 5 percent of the population according to some reports. And in honor of the most famous, though fictitious sufferer, the overwhelming urge for a midnight snack is nicknamed Dagwood syndrome.

Beyond questions about sleep disorders and their causes is the greater mystery of sleep itself. Although the fundamental reason we sleep is still a matter of intense research, there is no debate about the fact that a good night's sleep is key to feeling healthy; and that problems getting regular, restful sleep comprise one of the most common sources of health complaints.

## The Emergency Room

Dr. House's patients frequently enter through the emergency room after suddenly collapsing, suffering a seizure, or some other attack that strikes like a lightning bolt from clear skies. For instance, in "Babies and Bathwater" (1-18), a young woman who is pregnant suddenly becomes disoriented while driving. After she pulls the car over, she collapses. Then she's in the hospital, surrounded by Dr. House's team.

When someone goes to an emergency room, the context is entirely different than that of an established primary care relationship. The physician and patient usually don't know each other at all. There may be few if any medical records on hand. The symptoms probably seem serious and urgent, at least to the patient.

"When I see a patient, no matter what the complaint, no matter how they look, good, bad, or indifferent, I look for and think about as many life-threatening causes as I can," says Richard O'Brien, M.D., an emergency physician in Scranton, Pennsylvania, who is a spokesman for the American College of Emergency Physicians.

When considering possible causes of symptoms in a patient in an emergency room, it is not just a matter of how common or rare a particular health threat may be. Unlike a family physician, who will likely check off the most common diseases first, an emergency physician ranks possible diagnoses by how fast they progress and their potential lethality.

"I start with the worst scenario. When you walk though the door and tell me you have chest pain, I don't even start with heart attack in my mind, I really don't. I start with thoracic dissection of the aorta, which is absolutely the worst thing you could have that could cause chest pain, because it could kill you in seconds. When somebody comes in with an infection, I don't think of pneumonia or urinary infection first, I think of life-threatening meningococcal meningitis: because my door says the word 'Emergency,'" Dr. O'Brien says. "We look for the thing that will kill you first, the thing that will maim you second, and then you take a deep breath and if you find another cause or you need to refer to a specialist or call in a consultant, you do that."

The types of presenting problems that typically come before an emergency physician are naturally those that seem to be more urgent than the symptoms that bring people to a primary care physician.

## COMMON PRESENTING PROBLEMS IN EMERGENCY MEDICINE

- Chest pain
- Difficulty breathing
- Abdominal pain
- Fever
- Cough
- Injuries
- Loss of consciousness

Almost half the patients featured on *House, M.D.* arrive at the hospital after collapsing, suffering a seizure, or suffering a stroke. At real emergency departments across the nation, about 14 percent of patients arrive by ambulance. About one in 100 patients who come to emergency departments is unconscious or requires immediate resuscitation.

The more dramatic the symptoms a patient has when presenting in the emergency department, the more straightforward the diagnosis and treatment may be.

"When they come in horribly ill or terribly injured, I don't want to say it's easy, but intellectually it is, your hand is forced. When somebody comes in with a life-threatening ventricular tachycardia rhythm in the heart, I get paddles out and shock them. There's no discussion. It's done," says Dr. O'Brien. "However, when you come in and you are weak and dizzy and you've been that way for years and I'm the fortieth doctor to take a crack at this, that's difficult."

Physicians listen to what patients say, but the patients' bodies also "speak."

"It's very hard to fake sweating, if you are in a normal temperature room. If you are in a room where you really shouldn't be sweating and you are, then you are sick. If you are in a normal temperature room and your skin is cool and clammy, you're sick. I don't know what it is yet. Maybe it's your blood sugar. Maybe you are septic. Maybe you are a young woman who just had a ruptured ovarian artery from an ectopic pregnancy. I don't know yet, but I figure there is something wrong," Dr. O'Brien says.

"If you aren't mentating right, something's wrong. I had a college student come in. She was an English major. She should be eloquent, but isn't mentating right. You ask her a question and she says, 'Where's my purse? What happened?' I say, 'I don't know. The police just brought you in. Does anything hurt?' And she says, 'Well, I have a little headache. But where's my purse?' And she keeps saying that, then I know something's not right."

Emergency physicians in the United States often face more unknowns than their colleagues in other countries. That's because the U.S. health care system is so fragmented, with independent providers who can't easily share information. When a patient arrives at an emergency room, the physician on duty may have no information about the patient's medical history. By contrast, in Sweden 90 percent of general practitioners maintain electronic medical records on their patients.

According to an international survey performed by the Commonwealth Fund, the United States lags behind other English-speaking nations. Compared to Australia, Canada, New Zealand, and the United Kingdom, the United States scored worst on both the percentage of patients that were sent for duplicate tests by different health care professionals and worst in terms of not having medical records or test results reach a doctor's office in time for an appointment. The proponents of electronic medical records say that they could help close such information gaps.

U.S. Senator Bill Frist, M.D., wrote an article in favor of better electronic medical records systems. "Americans should be able to access their records wherever they go. This ranks as a high priority, because existing systems like the VA's are useless outside of the organizations that build them. If two travelers get into a car accident a thousand miles from home, the emergency room they arrive at should be able to access a system that can bring up their full medical history, their allergies, and information about the medications they take. Right now, in fact, outdated government regulations stop many hospitals from setting up systems that would do this."

Of course bringing medical records into the twenty-first century will require a substantial investment, not just in terms of money but also in redesigning how health care professionals go about their work. A report from the Institute of Medicine (IOM), while arguing strongly in favor of using information technology to improve health care quality, included warnings, too.

"Although computerized information systems have tremendous potential for improving information management, such systems are often underused or implemented in such a way that they increase the workload on caregivers and staff. This is counterproductive and should be avoided," the IOM report stated.

The effort to use technology to give physicians more information to go on when a new patient presents to them is just one of the changes occurring in front-line medical practice.

## Ambulances

The emergency physician's job is a bit different when patients arrive at the hospital by ambulance.

An old nickname for an ambulance is a "meat wagon." The slang term fit when ambulances were just trucks or station wagons modified so that a stretcher could fit inside. Today some ambulances can be likened to rolling emergency rooms. They are packed with sophisticated equipment and staffed with highly trained paramedics or other emergency medical technicians. Crews of advanced life support ambulances do much more than simply pick up and deliver patients; they begin the process of diagnosis and even treatment well before the patient reaches the hospital.

Guidelines for heart attack treatment call for first responders to be able to use electrocardiograms to diagnose a heart attack and properly use a defibrillator to shock a heart back into normal rhythm. Automatic defibrillators are taking things a step further, allowing people with little or no training to restart a victim's heartbeat.

Making a diagnosis in the field can save critical minutes, allowing hospitals to alert staff, prepare cardiology labs or operating rooms, and begin treatment as soon as the patient arrives. A study of hospitals that showed the greatest success in reducing treatment times for patients needing emergency angioplasty treatment after a heart attack showed that key steps included equipping and training ambulance crews to perform electrocardiograms in the field . . . and then relying on the reports from ambulance crews to activate treatment teams before the patient arrived at the hospital.

The trend toward extending diagnosis and treatment into the "pre-hospital" arena is continuing with some hospital systems training their paramedics to give drugs that can break open blood clots that cause heart attacks.

"They see chest pain all day long. A good, seasoned paramedic pretty much can tell you how sick the patient is. When they call me on the radio to get medical orders for something, I pipe right up, because if they need me, there is something seriously wrong with the patient," Dr. O'Brien says.

Sometimes the actual presentation of a patient to a health care professional is now coming after diagnosis and treatment, not before. Perhaps the most dramatic example is the growing use of automatic external defibrillators, or AEDs. These devices can diagnose ventricular fibrillation in a person who has collapsed with sudden cardiac arrest and then deliver powerful electrical shocks to kick the fluttering heart back into normal rhythm. AEDs require little training to use. They can literally talk people through the procedure with voice prompts. They are being used by flight attendants aboard aircraft, coaches at high school sports events, and many others.

An AED might have come in handy in "Heavy" (1-16). A ten-year-old collapses during gym class. The gym teacher realizes her heart has stopped pumping blood and calls 911. If the gym had been equipped with an AED, he could have tried shocking the girl's heart right away, without having to wait for paramedics to arrive. An increasing number of schools are buying AEDs, which cost a little more than $1,000 each. Some states even require that schools or fitness facilities install AEDs . . . just in case.

One of the most successful deployments of AEDs has been in Las Vegas casinos. An analysis of a series of 105 cases of people collapsing with ventricular fibrillation in casinos showed that slightly more than half survived to be discharged from a hospital. That survival rate is far higher than typical for people struck by sudden cardiac arrest in general.

Time is absolutely critical in these cases, because the quivering heart cannot pump blood to the patient's brain. In the casino experience, security personnel were able to attach an AED to the patient within an average of three and a half minutes after witnessing a collapse. By comparison, it took an average of almost ten minutes for the first paramedics to arrive on the scene. Undoubtedly, that six-minute difference was vital to the successful resuscitation of many patients. Indeed, three out of four patients survived when they were shocked back into normal heart rhythm within three minutes.

Later in this book, we will look at other examples of how computer technology is stepping in to perform tasks that were once solely the province of physicians.

## Communication

Of course, patients and physicians need to be able to communicate well in order to efficiently move from presentation to treatment. However, they may not always be speaking the same language; that is, a word that means one specific thing to a doctor may mean something different to the patient. That can be true even for a simple word such as fever.

For example, a survey of parents who brought their children to an emergency department in Cincinnati found that although most of them knew that a fever means the body temperature is elevated, they did not connect that general definition to specific body temperatures. For instance, the researchers wrote that parents might say that their child has had a fever for several days, but not specify that the body temperature was 102 degrees for the first days, but only 99 degrees for the last few days. The additional detail can make a difference in how physicians decide to respond.

The survey also indicated that while the parents generally knew the meaning of terms like diarrhea and constipation, they differed on details that could be important to a physician. Most of the parents could not accurately define meningitis, lethargy, or virus. The researchers who did the study said physicians need to make sure exactly what parents mean, even with seemingly simple medical terms.

Naturally the communication barrier is more extreme when physician and patients really don't speak the same language or come from different cultures. Multilingual and multicultural disconnects have always occurred, but they are becoming more common as communities become more diverse.

Almost one out of five people in the United States speaks a language other than English at home. Most of them speak Spanish, but there are over 300 languages spoken across the nation. According to the federal government, the most common languages after English and Spanish are French, German, Italian, Chinese, Tagalog, Polish, Korean, Vietnamese, Portuguese, Japanese, Greek, Arabic, Hindi, Russian, Yiddish, Thai, Persian, French Creole, and Armenian.

Dr. House and his colleagues rarely encounter patients who don't speak English fluently, even though responses to the 2000 U.S. Census indicate that almost a million people in New Jersey have at least some trouble speaking English. Language issues play a minor role in the episode "Humpty Dumpty" (2-03). The patient, who does some manual labor for Dr. Cuddy, speaks Spanish better than English. His little brother, who is not yet in high school, steps in to do some informal translation at the hospital.

Federal regulations require that any physician who accepts federal funds (which includes doctors who treat patients covered by Medicare or Medicaid) take steps to serve patients with limited English skills. These steps may include hiring translators who are either in the exam room or on the telephone with both the doctor and patient.

Because hiring a professional translator can seem like a burden to a physician, some have used friends or family of patients as informal translators, just as the Princeton-Plainesboro doctors do in "Humpty Dumpty." However, that practice does not always work well. Information may be left out or shaded in ways that make it harder for the doctor to understand the patient's complaint or to provide advice on testing and treatment. In some cases, children who speak English have been used as translators for their non-English-speaking parents. Just imagine the difficult task faced by a twelve-year-old boy forced into translating his mother's complaints about a gynecological problem.

One study found that "ad hoc interpretation," that is, using office staff or other people who happen to be available, but are not trained interpreters, often led to misinterpretations. Up to half the words and phrases used were incorrectly interpreted. What's more, ad hoc interpreters hear patient medical information that is supposed to be kept private between the patient and provider.

Culture itself can interfere with communication between a patient and physician. Here's how the Institute of Medicine report *Unequal Treatment* described hypothetical encounters between a white physician and a Latino or white middle-aged man who were both having symptoms that might be related to heart problems:

"Suppose the Latino and the white patient both experience exactly the same symptoms and describe their pain to the doctor. Will the doctor come to the same clinical decision for the Latino and the white? Expression of pain symptoms differs among cultural and racial groups. White doctors may simply understand pain reports better from members of their own racial group. When the white male talks to the doctor, the doctor relates easily to the patient's report; when the Latino tells his story, the doctor follows less well, and picks up fewer implicit clues," the report states.

As a result, even when there is no bias or prejudice on the part of the physician, the two patients presenting with the same symptoms may be referred for different tests because of cultural differences that affect patient-physician communication.

When patients first present themselves, physicians are trained to look first for the most common or most dangerous possible conditions. These are the cases that are dealt with routinely, and thus would never reach Dr. House. He wants to treat only the "zebras."

## Zebras

Ask physicians about the last time they saw a zebra and almost all will know you aren't inquiring about a trip to the zoo or an African safari. In the medical world, a zebra is that strange case that strolls in every now and then, breaking the routine and proving again that all the laws of probability do not rule out the improbable.

Some zebras are immediately perplexing, resisting categorization. Others display the signs and symptoms of a mundane complaint . . . and only later reveal their true stripes.

Being a zebra is not usually good for a patient. It can mean trekking along a crooked trail of physicians and clinics . . . being told nothing is wrong or being treated for the wrong diagnosis or being saddled with frustrating and fearsome uncertainty. For physicians, zebras can be frustrating, even maddening, but they are also fascinating. Zebras punctuate the routine. They present a challenge, a worthy opponent . . . something that mundane microbes and chronic complaints cannot offer. Indeed, one synonym for a medical zebra combines the word fascination with -oma, the suffix meaning tumor, to produce "fascinoma."

The character of Gregory House embodies, in the extreme, that fascination with peculiar cases. John Sotos, M.D., has known the attraction of medical zebras since his first year of medical school, when he heard the standard caution against thinking of exotic African animals when hearing hoofbeats while strolling on an American street. In spite of that warning, indeed intrigued by it, he began collecting zebras, jotting down their key features on what became "Zebra Cards." Eventually, Dr. Sotos published a book of his Zebra Cards, in order to help fellow physicians keep their minds open to surprising possibilities as they catalogue the symptoms of their patients.

To Dr. Sotos, surprise is the key feature of a medical zebra. Being rare is not enough. For instance, if a child of a patient with an extremely rare genetic disease also developed the disease, no one would be particularly surprised. The case would not be a zebra, even if it were a one-in-a-million occurrence.

A common condition can also be a zebra. Each year over a million people in the United States suffer a heart attack. If the symptoms are crushing pain in the chest or left arm, there is no element of surprise. However, Dr. Sotos notes that there are a dozen documented cases in which a headache was the only complaint mentioned by a person who, it turned out, actually had had a heart attack; now that's a zebra.

Headaches can also be caused by brain tumors, though of course only an extremely tiny percentage of headaches signal brain tumors.

Is that a zebra? Well, if so, the stripes are pretty thin. Few doctors are going to suspect a brain tumor right away, but as time passes and other explanations fall by the wayside, then brain tumor may rise to the top of the list. But since brain tumor may have been somewhere down the list—and perhaps high up on the patient's personal list of feared diagnoses—it isn't a strong zebra candidate.

Zebras are so familiar to physicians and medical students that it seems the term has always been part of medical lingo. Who coined the term? Dr. Sotos says he searched for twenty years, and finally concluded that the best claim belonged to the late Theodore E. Woodward, M.D., who taught at the University of Maryland School of Medicine in Baltimore for nearly fifty years. Dr. Woodward was also nominated for a Nobel Prize, and received an award from President Franklin D. Roosevelt, for his role in developing treatments for typhus and typhoid fever.

Dr. Sotos says that beginning in the 1940s Dr. Woodward admonished his medical students, "Don't look for zebras on Greene Street," referring to the street outside the University of Maryland medical school. Over time, the advice became more general: "When you hear hoofbeats behind you, don't expect to see a zebra."

Dr. Woodward died in 2005 at the age of ninety-one, but his counsel to young doctors endures. And it gives a handle to the search at the heart of every episode of *House, M.D.*, where hoofbeats are interesting only if they might signal something other than a horse. As Dr. House said in the pilot, "Let's find out what kind of zebra we're dealing with here."

# TWO

# Poking and Probing

**M**ost of the physical examinations seen on *House, M.D.* take place during the vignettes in the clinic that Dr. House works so hard to avoid. On the show, these cameo appearances are often played for laughs. In one case, a woman had confused strawberry jelly and spermicidal jelly. In another, Dr. House hinted to a young patient with a cold that he might need a lung transplant, in order to frighten him into signing up for health care coverage.

The clinic exam room scenes may be just little asides from the main story line, but they briefly encapsulate key features of typical office visits. The patient explains why he or she came to the doctor's office, known as the "chief complaint." Then the doctor's questions begin to bring out details of the "history of the present illness." During this question-and-answer exchange, there is an important balance between zeroing in on the patient's symptoms and surveying the whole body for clues the patient may not even realize are connected.

"With some people you just focus in on one thing. If they have a rash, you just look at the rash. But you still have to keep the entire patient in mind, because maybe they also have joint problems," Dr. Rick Kellerman says, noting that other related problems may influence the ultimate diagnosis.

In "Sleeping Dogs Lie" (2-18), failure to follow up on a rash delayed the diagnosis. The patient's chief complaint was being unable to sleep. A rash she had noticed earlier seemed irrelevant. It wasn't.

In order to be thorough, physicians do what's called a review of systems, which is a method for quickly checking the body's organs and other parts. The review of systems moves the discussion toward specific queries intended to bring out pieces of information that the patient may not think are relevant or noteworthy.

Questions in the review of systems may include:

- "Have you had any headaches?"

- "How's your vision?"

- "Have you been coughing?"

- "How's your appetite?"

- "Any aching joints?"

- "Any swelling in your feet or ankles?"

The review often goes from head to toe . . . as does the actual physical examination that follows. And the questions are also grouped by organ system. Questions related to allergies and the immune system tend to go together, as do questions about neurological and psychiatric aspects of the patient's health.

All of these questions are part of building the patient's medical history, the important context of the current chief complaint. But the questions are not just about how the patient is doing that day. The physician also needs to know about the past, about the patient's family and work and social life, all of which have profound influences on overall health and the specific issues of the moment.

Despite his pronouncement that "Everybody lies," Dr. House relies heavily on talking to patients about what is going on in their lives, in order to put the signs and symptoms in context. In one episode, Dr. House notices the patient is wearing new eyeglasses and recently had her teeth whitened. So when she presses him for urgent action on a cold she had a week earlier, he surmises that she is trying to take advantage of all the health care benefits she can before she leaves her job. In the first episode, a clinic patient's skin was orange from eating large amounts of carrots and taking niacin supplements. But Dr. House also diagnosed a failing marriage, since the patient's wife hadn't seemed to care that the man's skin had taken an odd new hue.

---

### Symptoms and Signs

Symptoms are what a patient complains of.

Signs are what the physician finds in the exam.

---

There is a theme and order common to most modern physical examinations, with variations depending on the reason for the visit. Often before the patient and physician meet, a nurse checks the patient's vital signs and weight. The four vital signs are pulse, blood pressure, temperature, and respiration.

## The "Fifth" Vital Sign

Some experts and institutions are calling pain the fifth vital sign and urging health care professionals to routinely ask patients about it. Pain is not always obvious. Patients with chronic pain may become adept at concealing it, though it may reveal itself in the pattern of breathing, the manner of walking, the way the patient holds himself.

The Joint Commission on Accreditation of Healthcare Organizations has standards for pain management that hospitals and other institutions are expected to meet:

"Pain can be a common part of the patient experience; unrelieved pain has adverse physical and psychological effects. The patient's right to pain management is respected and supported. The health care organization plans, supports, and coordinates activities and resources to assure the pain of all patients is recognized and addressed appropriately."

Dr. House would probably agree that assessing pain should be a routine part of any exam and then addressing the pain should be a high priority.

---

With information from the history and vital signs in hand, the physician begins physically inspecting the patient, poking and prodding to get the body to reveal its secrets.

"And I refer to that as a dance, where you look at the ears, throat, neck, thyroid, heart, lungs. I tend to go from top to bottom. I tell medical students that it's a dance and they have to learn the dance," Dr. Kellerman says.

Robert B. Taylor, M.D., at the Oregon Health & Science University (OSHU) in Portland, Oregon, who edited the *Manual of Family Practice*, points out a couple of reasons for the top-to-bottom routine. First, by going in the same order every time and not skipping around, the physician is less likely to forget things. Second, it seems more socially comfortable for most patients to start by looking at the head, eyes, ears, and so on. And usually "top to bottom" actually means head to toe . . . and then lastly to the "bottom." After a pelvic, genital, and rectal exam, most people understandably are ready for the exam to end.

"Examining the head is the least threatening and intrusive part, so we start there and work down," Dr. Taylor says.

When a patient has a clear and specific complaint, for instance, "My knee hurts," it makes sense to take shortcuts. Indeed, a patient complaining about a foot problem would probably be befuddled by a doctor who insisted on starting with an eye examination. But when a patient is new to a physician or has a general or diffuse complaint, such as fatigue, a thorough going-over is useful. For the type of puzzling cases that Dr. House and his colleagues see, a complete and scrupulous end-to-end examination would frequently make sense. And sometimes one clue takes the case in an entirely new direction.

When physicians look at and into the eyes of patients, among the things they want to know are the following: Do they move properly? Are the whites really white? How do the pupils react to light? How does the back of the eye look when viewed through an ophthalmoscope?

In "Babies and Bathwater" (1-18), a subtle drooping of one eyelid indicated a possible neurological issue. The examination led the team to suspect a paraneoplastic syndrome; specifically, Lambert-Eaton myasthenic syndrome, which pointed toward a lung tumor.

---

## Paraneoplastic Syndromes

In several episodes, neurological problems, such as passing out while driving, a seizure, numbness in the arms, and respiratory arrest, led to a cancer diagnosis. It's called paraneoplastic syndrome or paraneoplastic neurological disorder.

## Poking and Probing

Paraneoplastic neurological disorders are specifically those syndromes that involve an autoimmune attack that, while intended to fight the tumor, ends up damaging nerve cells. This sort of collateral damage is apparently caused by antigens on the surfaces of nerve cells that may look similar to those on the cancer cells.

In other episodes, paraneoplastic syndromes are included in the list of possible diagnoses of cases with neurological symptoms. They should be, according to cancer experts, who estimate that less than one out of 100 cancer patients will have a paraneoplastic neurological disorder. That doesn't sound like much, and indeed it means these syndromes are far less common than other cancer-related problems, but with over 1.3 million cases of cancer in the United Sates each year, that rate means that perhaps 10,000 Americans develop paraneoplastic neurological disorders every year.

The rates vary dramatically depending on the type of underlying cancer. Paraneoplastic syndromes are seen in up to 3 percent of patients with small-cell lung cancer, as depicted in "Babies and Bathwater." But less than one in a thousand women with gynecologic cancers will also have to deal with a paraneoplastic syndrome.

The syndromes can be hard to pin down. They are not usually detected through standard tests of blood or cerebrospinal fluid, or through MRI scans. But if the standard tests rule out other possible causes for the symptoms, then paraneoplastic neurological disorder may remain a possibility. A firm diagnosis may depend on finding the underlying tumor or detecting antibodies that are attacking the patient's nerve cells.

Paraneoplastic syndromes are more important than the plain numbers might suggest because they are frequently the first sign of cancer in the patient. Unfortunately, even if the underlying tumor is treated successfully, the neurological damage may be permanent, leaving the cancer survivor disabled.

Some studies indicate that cancer patients with paraneoplastic syndromes fare better than other cancer patients. It may be that the early warning given by the paraneoplastic symptoms means that doctors can catch the tumor before it progresses too far to treat.

However, the higher average length of survival may be a mirage. It may be that the paraneoplastic syndromes bring patients to the attention of physicians earlier in the course of the cancer. This "lead-time bias," as it is known, means that more time passes between the date of the diagnosis and the date of death when the cancer is fatal; but rather than the death occurring later, what is really happening is that the diagnosis just occurred earlier.

---

Now back to the physical exam. After the eyes, doctors look at the ears, into the ear canal, and at the eardrum. Perhaps they do a simple hearing test.

"I used to use a wristwatch," Dr. Taylor says. "But now wristwatches don't tick anymore! So I'll just make a little noise by rubbing my fingers together. It's a quick-and-dirty screening test."

Nose: Look up inside the nose with a light. Perhaps do a more complete inspection, if there are indications of sinusitis.

A toddler's strange breathing sounds tipped off Dr. House to take a closer look up the boy's nose in "Mob Rules" (1-15). The patient's brother said the toddler was wheezing, but Dr. House was more specific: The sound was a whistling in the boy's upper airways or nose. Following the whistle, Dr. House reached up the nostril with tweezers to extract a tiny toy policeman.

Mouth: Inspect the tongue, teeth, salivary glands, and the back of the throat.

Neck: How well does the neck move? How does the thyroid gland look and feel?

## Poking and Probing

In "Three Stories" (1-21), Cameron checked the thyroid of a high school volleyball player. What might seem a bit odd about that inspection is that the patient's chief complaint was knee pain. But Cameron was being thorough and it paid off. She found a nodule on the girl's thyroid. Thyroid dysfunction can cause both mental issues and joint pain. The neck exam also includes checking the carotid artery, listening for a sound called a "bruit" (pronounced BROO-ee). Bruit is a French word that simply means "noise." The medical meaning in this case is a sound of turbulence in blood flow that may indicate either a narrowing in the blood vessel or its opposite: an aneurysm.

In the episode "Love Hurts" (1-20), Chase heard a small bruit in the carotid artery of the patient. He speculated it could indicate an aneurysm caused by trauma. Although Dr. House dismissed the clue at first, later on it became clear the patient had endured physical abuse.

Chest: Do both sides of the chest move equally as the patient takes a deep breath? Tap the chest to compare the sound from one side to the other. Clear lungs resonate. A dull tap sound may indicate fluid or a mass in the lungs. Listen to the lungs with a stethoscope. Coarse, rough sounds, called rhonchi, are a sign of bronchitis. Rales, which sound like wind whistling through leaves, are characteristic of pneumonia.

Rales, decreased breath sounds, or a wheeze are also signs of asthma. If the sound has a single tone, the obstruction is probably in just one area, while polyphonic sounds indicate more generalized obstruction. Dr. House used such breath sounds and other clues from a clinic exam to determine that a patient's mother had been cutting back on the boy's asthma medication.

Heart: There are five key things to listen for—four valves and along the sternum in the middle of the chest. A very coarse heart murmur may even be felt by hand. Tapping around the heart can indicate its size. The heart and chest examination may be repeated with the patient lying down.

Lymph nodes: Check for swelling under the arm.

Breast exam: In female patients, feel for any lumps and look for other abnormalities in the breast.

Breasts figured prominently in a clinic sidebar during "Fidelity" (1-07). The patient's chief complaint was shortness of breath. Dr. House listened to her chest with a stethoscope, asked about heart disease in her family, and ordered an EKG to check her heartbeat. Then he noticed her rather large breast implants.

In this case, the implants did not turn out to be the cause of the patient's symptoms. Implants do raise questions for both women and their physicians, when it comes to screening for breast cancer. One journal article on recommendations for clinical breast examinations noted that some physicians are uncertain about how implants might affect their ability to detect breast lumps. However, the authors pointed out that since implants are placed behind a woman's natural breast tissue, the steps used to perform a clinical breast examination are exactly the same as those used in women without breast implants.

Implants can be a challenge for radiologists trying to detect small breast lumps on mammograms. In general, experts recommend additional images be taken during the mammography process, in order to compensate for the fact that the silicone or saline in breast implants tends to block X-rays.

Abdomen: Inspect. Tap and feel to estimate size and condition of the liver and spleen. Listen to bowel sounds.

Legs: Look for signs of good circulation, for instance the quality of the skin of the feet.

Neurological: With the patient again sitting up, a check of how the muscles move in the face, head, and upper body can offer hints about the health of nerves in the head. Check reflexes: the "knee-jerk" test with a rubber hammer tapping the knee to produce an automatic response from the spinal cord. The rubber hammer is also used to gently stroke the outer soles of the feet. A normal response is for the toes to curl. Little or no response to these tests may indicate nerve damage from disease or trauma.

Then, near the end of the physical exam, come the pelvic examination for women and a hernia and genital area check for men. And finally the rectal exam, including a prostate exam in men.

## Smell Check

While the senses of sight, touch, and hearing usually get the most work during a physical examination, smell can also play an important role. Writing in the *New England Journal of Medicine*, a young physician named Andrew Bomback, M.D., noted recently that although he seems to spend less and less time examining patients and more and more time looking at test results and imaging reports, one part of the physical exam cannot be replaced by tests: the patient's smell. The smell of dressings from a diabetic patient immediately reveals whether antibiotics may be needed to fight a wound infection. A patient's breath can warn of kidney problems. And of course, the aroma of cigarette smoke is a red flag of higher risks to both the immediate and long-term health of the patient.

## Cigarettes as Therapy

In "Damned If You Do" (1-05), a shopping mall Santa comes to the clinic, and Dr. House makes a point of sniffing the air as he enters the exam room. It turns out that the patient is pleading for effective treatment of his inflammatory bowel disease . . . which has led to unpleasant consequences with a lap full of kids . . . and the pungent odor that Dr. House recognized.

House writes a prescription for cigarettes. Two each day. He says studies have shown cigarette smoking is one of the most effective ways to control inflammatory bowel. Well, close, but no cigar. Studies have indeed shown that smokers are less likely to develop a type of inflammatory bowel disease known as ulcerative colitis, but smokers are more likely than nonsmokers to have Crohn's disease, which is another form of inflammatory bowel disease. Some studies indicate that rather than protecting people against ulcerative colitis, smoking just makes it more likely that people who are predisposed to either form of inflammatory bowel disease end up with the Crohn's disease form.

As for prescribing cigarettes to calm inflammatory bowel symptoms, it's definitely not mainstream practice. Based on hints of an effect, there have been studies of nicotine treatment for people with inflammatory bowel disease, but neither cigarettes nor nicotine patches are considered strong options. The main drug treatments include anti-inflammatory drugs and medicines that suppress the immune system. Other drugs are used to control symptoms.

The final, drastic option for some patients with severe disease may be surgery to remove the troublesome bowel.

When Wilson questions Dr. House's cigarette prescription, because smoking causes lung cancer, House remarks that there's no ribbon for lung cancer, because people blame smokers and think they deserve to die. Although the remark is a typical House zinger, it does contain some truth. A panel of lung cancer experts commissioned by the National Cancer Institute concluded that the stigma of smoking is one of the key reasons there is relatively little research into lung cancer treatments. Indeed, the federal government spends far more on breast cancer research than on lung cancer research, even though lung cancer is the leading cancer killer of both women and men in the United States.

However, House was wrong about the ribbons. Some lung cancer advocacy groups use ribbons that are clear plastic or crystal, in part to

symbolize the "invisibility" of the number-one cancer killer. So lung cancer ribbons do indeed exist . . . it's just that few people display them.

---

The rhythm of the physical examination is one of the fundamental skills that every physician must master.

"It's all orchestrated. The patient isn't jumping on and off the table.
It all goes very smoothly. The whole exam can be done in fifteen minutes or maybe a little longer if it includes a pelvic examination. Fifteen
minutes is routine with an experienced examiner," Dr. Taylor says.

Of course, physicians just beginning their careers take a bit longer
to run through everything. Dr. Taylor says that young physicians learn
the rhythm of the physical exam so that they do not leave out anything
and they aren't jumping back and forth, asking patients to sit up and lie
down again and again. Then after they become comfortable with the
full physical, physicians learn what they should focus on and what they
can leave out, based on the history the patient has provided. Editing
down the physical examination is a critical skill, because there simply is
not enough time to give each and every patient full head-to-toe scrutiny.

"The physical exam will depend on how focused their symptoms
are. If a patient comes in and says, 'Doctor, for the past three days I've
had back pain and burning when I pass my urine,' I'm not going to get
anything out of listening to their heart or their lungs; that's not their
problem. Nor do I need to do a screening neurological examination. I
know that this almost certainly has to do with kidney, bladder, and
urinary tract. I can focus the exam there," Dr. Taylor points out.

"On the other hand, if they come in with a general symptom,
things like tiredness and fatigue, weight loss, that kind of thing, or
they come up with an unexpected sign, for instance, they are found
to be anemic, perhaps after donating blood, without having been
aware of the anemia; then these situations call for a much more

thorough examination, because the list of possibilities is not only much longer, it can be more ominous, like cancer."

Patients have a right to check that their physician performed enough of a physical examination to understand the problem.

"Sometimes in a busy day there is a tendency to underexamine the patient. It's okay for the patient to ask, 'Have you done everything? Have you examined all the areas you need to examine?'" Dr. Taylor says.

And on the doctor's part, a final question loops back around to the open-ended beginning of the visit: "Anything else?" As complete as the history and physical examination may have been, it is not uncommon for patients to keep something inside. Then just as they are leaving, out it comes.

It's sometimes called the "doorknob question," because patients may blurt out a withheld concern as they or the doctor have a hand on the doorknob on the way out of the exam room. In "The Mistake" (2-08), Chase recalled thinking the patient might have had a doorknob question because of the way she hesitated when he sent her on her way after a brief conversation. Later it turned out he had indeed failed to properly follow up on clues of a serious problem.

A doorknob question may be something the patient is embarrassed about or a symptom that seems irrelevant to the main topic of that particular visit. Patients who are elderly or have chronic illnesses may hold something back, in part because they may be reluctant to dump a long laundry list of concerns on the doctor. In one study, one out of five patients raised a new problem at the end of the office visit.

While eliminating doorknob questions may be an unattainable dream for physicians, some experts say the best way to reduce the number of last-minute surprises—and the schedule disruptions they cause—is to do a better job of listening, and not interrupting, at the beginning of the visit. If patients are encouraged to bring up all their concerns, big or small, a single issue or several, early in the encounter, then perhaps they will be less likely to say, as the doctor is heading out to see the next patient, "Oh, by the way."

Dr. Taylor says that when he was first learning the ropes, he wasn't just thrown into examining patients. Medical students observe, and then repeat bits of the exam that their supervising physician has just demonstrated. Then they move up to doing part or all of the examination under supervision before going solo.

"It's gradual. Young doctors are not told to just suddenly go in and do it," he says. "But here at OHSU we have a curious program that we didn't have in my time. Before the incoming medical students have had even a single class, they have an opportunity to spend a week living in the home of a rural doctor, and go in to the hospital and office with that doctor. These kids are going to remember very clearly the first time they were sent into a room to help examine a patient, because all they've had is a day and a half crash course in what end of the stethoscope you put in your ears."

And speaking of that universal symbol of doctors, when stethoscopes first came into use almost two centuries ago, the low-tech assemblage of rubber tubes and metal was the leading edge of medical technology. French physician René Théophile Hyacinthe Laënnec is credited with creating and popularizing the stethoscope. The name comes from a Greek word for chest: *stethos*. The stethoscope's third century is a question mark, though, as ultrasound, CT, MRI, and computer programs threaten to replace tubing, chestpieces, eartips, and the physician's interpretation of the body's sounds. (See chapter 3 for more on the future of the stethoscope.)

The shift in technology also affects attitudes toward physical examination itself.

"The huge difference today is the attitude toward physical examination. The attitude today is, 'I don't really have to know this so much, because I'm going to pick it up on CT, MRI, and sophisticated blood tests. In my day we didn't have CT, we didn't have MRI, we didn't have these sophisticated blood tests. You depended a lot more on your eyes, ears, and intuition. You had to be really good at physical diagnosis. Today I think there is a sense in some corners that you can finesse it, because we'll pick things up on treadmill tests and imaging, etc. There is much more of a reliance on technology today than there was.

"I think it's a reality. I think it's kind of sad, though; because they are losing part of the art of medicine," Dr. Taylor says.

The "art of medicine" is one of those phrases that is frequently used, but only occasionally defined. Most physicians see it as that skill that clinicians must develop to integrate science, their clinical experience, and the understanding they have of the patient's wishes. It is an art, because while science is the essential underpinning of medicine, each patient and each encounter is unique and requires judgments tailored to that particular situation.

Dr. Taylor recalled an aphorism of the pioneering diagnostician, Sir William Osler: "Listen to the patient. He is telling you the diagnosis." And even with all the latest technology available, he says the general rule of thumb is that 60 to 70 percent of diagnoses are made based on just the history.

For example, a physician examining a patient with severe headaches that might be migraines may be tempted to order an MRI scan. But it turns out that three simple questions can sort out most cases:

Have your headaches

1. caused you to limit your activities?

2. Have they made you nauseous?

3. Are you noticeably bothered by light?

If the patient answers yes to all three questions, then there is a very high probability that the problem is migraine and nothing else.

---

## Sir William Osler, M.D.

One of the most influential figures in the development of modern diagnostic methods was Sir William Osler, M.D. Osler was born in the wilds of Ontario, Canada, on July 12, 1849. He helped set the foundations of medical education in the United States as one of the first instructors at the Johns Hopkins Hospital and School of Medicine in Baltimore, Maryland. During his tenure from 1888 to 1905, Osler helped push for hands-on education of young physicians.

"Medicine is learned by the bedside and not in the classroom," Osler preached.

Working with patients on the hospital wards may seem like an obvious way to learn medicine, but it was not the usual practice in U.S. medical schools of the time.

"Observe, record, tabulate, communicate. Use your five senses," and "The four points of a medical student's compass are: Inspection, Palpation, Percussion, and Auscultation" are two more of Osler's oft-repeated aphorisms about examining patients.

Pediatrician Billy Andrews, M.D., wrote about Osler's influence on today's physicians in the *Southern Medical Journal*.

Dr. Andrews wrote that, "[My dean] let me know that I was an academic grandchild of Sir William Osler, and must continue Osler's high ideals and practice. Many of the members of this society are also academic grandchildren, great grandchildren, and possibly even great, great grandchildren of Sir William Osler."

In 1891, Dr. Osler wrote *The Principles and Practice of Medicine*. It is considered such an important milestone in the medical literature that in 1999, the 150th anniversary of Osler's birth, the Johns Hopkins

University Department of Medicine created the Osler Textbook Room in the very spot where the doctor wrote his textbook.

Dr. Osler might have looked favorably on Dr. House's ability to observe and diagnose his patients, but he probably would not have liked House's sour attitude.

"[I]t is an unpardonable mistake to go about among patients with a long face," Dr. Osler said in one oft-quoted speech.

---

Of course, even when a skilled physician asks all the right questions and pokes, prods, and listens to all the right body parts, some patient complaints are left unresolved.

"It's very important for a family physician, a primary care physician, to know where their limits are. Ninety-five percent of the stuff that comes in you can take care of. Even the rare and bizarre one you can usually take care of. But there are other times when you just can't figure it out," says Dr. Rick Kellerman.

"I had one lady that I just could not figure out what was going on with her. So I sent her to a neurologist," he recalls.

There was a medical student in the office that afternoon. Dr. Kellerman remembers telling the student that it seems in most cases when he refers a patient to a specialist, because he can't figure out what's wrong, the specialist won't figure it out either.

"Right at that moment, the phone rang. I picked it up. It was the neurologist. He said, 'You know what, I can't figure out what's going on with this lady,'" Dr. Kellerman says.

## Going Beyond the Patient's Body

Most of the featured cases on *House, M.D.* are well past the overall survey of the typical physical exam. In any case, Dr. House usually leaves physical examination of patients to others.

## Poking and Probing

Physical examinations of patients are less common on the series than in most medical practices, but Dr. House and his team frequently investigate the physical surroundings of patients, their homes and offices. They have searched refrigerators, examined herbal teas, checked homemade tomato sauces, sought out traveling companions to ask questions and perform exams. They've looked everywhere for clues, including under the kitchen sink.

In real life, doctors rely on what patients tell them about their surroundings and possible exposures to microbes or toxins. With a waiting room or hospital ward full of patients, doctors just don't have time to take field trips to examine the physical environments of their patients.

Nevertheless, in cases of infectious disease outbreaks or toxic exposures, environmental investigations are critical to determining the source of the threat. While a patient's personal physician does not run out to test food for bacteria or clothes closets for signs of pesticide contamination, physician reports do trigger action by other health professionals from local, state, or federal public health agencies.

In 2001, the Epidemic Intelligence Service (EIS) of the U.S. Centers for Disease Control and Prevention celebrated a half century of training disease detectives to track down health threats at home and around the world. The EIS was established during the Korean War. The first class had just a couple of dozen students, but now more than 2,500 disease detectives have graduated from the two-year program.

EIS investigators often are stationed at local public health agencies and help out with the routine work of tracking local health issues and other public health duties. But whenever an outbreak occurs they are ready to swing into action to find the source of the illness. The problem may be as mundane as potato salad left out too long at a family reunion or a common microbe spreading diarrhea through a day-care center. But every now and then, EIS field agents confront medical puzzles that Dr. House would drool over.

45

Cryptosporidium that spread through the water supply sickened more than 400,000 people in Milwaukee, Wisconsin, in the spring of 1993. EIS agents supported local public health agencies to track down the source of the massive outbreak.

More than two dozen veterans suddenly developed respiratory problems and then died after attending an American Legion convention in Philadelphia in 1976. Working with local officials in Pennsylvania and in the home areas of the victims, EIS agents were part of an eight-month-long search. They hit one dead end after another. Cases seemed to be clustered in a convention hotel. But apparently not all the victims had been in the hotel. The common link eluded investigators as the death toll mounted. Eventually a type of waterborne bacterium was identified as the killer. It was dubbed Legionella pneumophila. After the Philadelphia outbreak, public health investigators found that this type of bacteria can grow in hot tubs, cooling towers used for air-conditioning, and other sources of water used for drinking or washing. People with weakened immune systems, the elderly, smokers, those with other diseases, are most at risk of developing serious consequences from infection with Legionella pneumophilia.

Most health problems are most serious for the oldest and youngest in our communities, as well as those with chronic illnesses. Of course, most of the patients on *House, M.D.* are young and otherwise healthy. That's one of the reasons their cases are so intriguing. But in 1993, young, healthy men and women began dying in New Mexico. In fact, it was the strong health of the victims that grabbed the interest of physicians.

A doctor checking on the sudden death of a young, championship-caliber long-distance runner was told the man had been on the way to attend the funeral of his twenty-one-year-old fiancée, who had died of similar symptoms. Both bride- and groom-to-be went from feeling fine to being unable to breathe in a matter of days. After local doctors raised the alarm, state public health experts and then EIS agents from the CDC moved in. The outbreak was one of the first times high-tech DNA tools were used to track an infectious agent during an outbreak. Within weeks, investigators on the scene and back at the CDC laboratories in Atlanta had gathered enough evidence to announce that the killer was a form of hantavirus, a pathogen that is common in deer mice. It had never been recognized as a virus that could sicken or kill people by attacking the lungs.

At the time, people wondered if perhaps the virus had recently mutated. But then doctors around the country checked samples saved from cases of unexplained deaths over the years. They found cases stretching back many years. In fact, the oldest known case dates back to 1959. What's more, local Navajo say there are ancient stories of young men dying suddenly in ways that seem similar to the modern cases of hantavirus infections. It may be that the virus has always been around, but was simply too uncommon to attract notice in most cases . . . and also too elusive to be identified before the development of DNA testing.

The hantavirus investigation began because doctors asked for help when they could not explain a cluster of unusual deaths. But some diseases must be reported, because of their potential to threaten public health. Reportable diseases include measles, whooping cough, gonorrhea, and salmonella infections. The reporting systems that are in place to identify such cases are examples of public health surveillance. Surveillance can flag outbreaks before they become big enough to overwhelm local hospitals and other health care institutions. But many public health experts warn that current surveillance methods are inadequate and might not catch the signs of a natural event or bioterror attack in time to prevent widespread illness, deaths, or panic.

The frequently haphazard nature of public health surveillance was illustrated in the *House, M.D.* episode "Poison" (1-08). A high school student got sick during a test and came to the hospital suffering nausea, disorientation, and a dangerously low heart rate. Then a second student was brought in with similar symptoms. Dr. House and his team quickly began looking for some connection between the two boys. But what if the second boy had been transported to a different hospital? Without centralized surveillance, the two cases might not have been linked, leaving doctors at a disadvantage.

One challenge of identifying outbreaks early is that the symptoms of many rare and potentially lethal conditions may look just like those of common and usually less serious ailments. In the hantavirus outbreak, the early symptoms were headache and fever. Without any specific test at the time, doctors didn't know whether a patient with apparently minor complaints that day might be dead the next. On the other hand, in the middle of cold and flu season, admitting every patient with aches and pains would quickly overwhelm any hospital.

Some public health agencies are beginning to harness the power of computers to help spot suspicious patterns. In 2005, North Carolina started using a system called the North Carolina Hospital Emergency Surveillance System to electronically link every hospital emergency department in the state. As patients are seen in an emergency room, their symptoms are entered into the hospital's computer system. Rather than just staying locked in that single system, key information about patient symptoms is regularly transmitted to a state public health computer. So if patients who got sick at the same place end up going to different hospitals, their cases would still be pooled together and compared to normal patterns of illness in the community.

As they unveiled the new alert system, officials noted that under the old system of reporting cases by manually sending in paper forms, it could take weeks to spot a disease outbreak. The hope is that with hospital computers automatically feeding information to the state database, unusual patterns caused by an epidemic or a bioterror attack will be noticed much more quickly. Indeed, officials told reporters at the news conference announcing the new surveillance system that just a week earlier it had helped public health officials respond within twenty-four hours to an outbreak of hepatitis A that originated with some contaminated food. They said before this system was created, they might not have connected the cases for weeks.

The North Carolina system is the first statewide program of its type, but the first elements of a national system are already taking shape. As one part of the long-term response to the anthrax attacks of 2001, the Centers for Disease Control and Prevention (CDC) is developing a national program, called BioSense, that will collect and analyze current illness reports from cities around the country. As with the North Carolina surveillance system, the purpose of BioSense is to spot unusual clusters of symptoms and illnesses within hours.

Of course, many people who don't feel well just stay home. These patients would not be detected by surveillance systems based in hospital emergency rooms, at least not until they become too ill to care for themselves. One idea for picking up spikes in illnesses in the community is to monitor sales of medicines in local pharmacies. National pharmacy chains already use sophisticated inventory control systems to track sales. There are both technical and legal hurdles that public health agencies would have to overcome before they could effectively plug in to commercial pharmacy computer systems. And then they would have to learn more about what is normal in the community, in order to reduce the number of false alarms. Nevertheless, a tracking system that analyzed sales of over-the-counter remedies and prescriptions phoned in by doctors might detect outbreaks well before people start crowding doctor's offices or emergency departments.

Every now and then, Dr. House sends Foreman, Chase, and Cameron to sneak into a patient's home to search for clues. Not only are such break-ins by individual physicians probably illegal, the secrecy probably would not be necessary. A physician can report suspicious cases to local public health authorities even if such reporting is not required. In general, public health authorities have the legal authority to search for clues or take other actions to protect the community.

Public health law in the United States dates back to the earliest days of the nation, when officials routinely inspected incoming sailing ships and quarantined any crews that showed symptoms of dangerous infectious diseases. State governors have varying degrees of authority to declare public health emergencies. They can order searches, quarantines, or even arrests in extreme cases. Such uses of police powers in the name of public health became rare in recent decades as infectious disease outbreaks dwindled due to the general improvement in the health of the population and mass vaccination campaigns.

However, the power to restrict individual liberty in the name of public health is occasionally invoked. In the early 1990s, rising rates of tuberculosis in a number of major cities prompted authorities to detain some patients. When tuberculosis patients don't complete a full course of therapy, which can include taking a number of different medicines for many months, the bacteria may become resistant to drug treatment. However, patients usually feel much better long before the treatment has killed all the tuberculosis bacteria in their bodies. Public health authorities in New York City and elsewhere worried that people who stopped treatment early and were carrying drug-resistant tuberculosis could create an epidemic of untreatable disease.

The New York City health commissioner issued orders that in certain cases patients should be detained in order to make sure they completed their tuberculosis therapy. In one study, among 8,000 patients with tuberculosis during a two-year period, 139 were detained during therapy. Another 150 were ordered to undergo "directly observed therapy." In these cases, rather than just being given pills and instructions on when to take them, the patients were told to report to a clinic where a staff person would watch them take their pills. Most of the time, small incentives, such as coupons for a fast-food meal were enough to get patients to report on schedule. But the threat of detention was there.

Of course, stepping on an individual's rights in order to protect the public health is considered to be ethical only when there is a good reason to believe that the forced treatment or other action is actually going to work. A recent systematic review of all the available studies on directly observed therapy for tuberculosis concluded that the strategy does not produce an important improvement in either the number of patients who complete their treatment or overall cure rates. The review by the Cochrane Collaboration looked at all known randomized controlled trials of directly observed therapy in both developing and developed nations. This scientific conclusion will likely have an impact on public health policy decisions about when tuberculosis patients should be required to accept treatment.

The effectiveness and ethics of mandatory treatment and other restrictions on individuals continues to be debated against a backdrop of concern about possible bioterror scenarios, including the use of smallpox virus or other microbes.

---

### "Phantoms"

Sometimes there is nothing to find . . . well, not really nothing, but no physical culprit, no microbe, no toxin. That's because some outbreaks of "temporary" mild illness may be a psychosomatic phenomenon, that is, the symptoms, nausea, headaches, fainting are quite real, but they likely are the result of the body reacting to a psychological impulse, rather than a physical pathogen.

Here's how investigators from the EIS summed up one incident at a high school: "In November 1998, a teacher noticed a 'gasoline-like' smell in her classroom, and soon thereafter she had a headache, nausea, shortness of breath, and dizziness. The school was evacuated, and eighty students and nineteen staff members went to the emergency room at the local hospital; thirty-eight persons were hospitalized overnight. Five days later, after the school had reopened, another seventy-one persons went to the emergency room."

Despite an extensive investigation by several government agencies, including the CDC's Epidemic Intelligence Service, no medical or environmental cause was found. However, the investigation did reveal important clues. The people who felt sick tended to be those who saw someone else who was ill, who knew a classmate was ill, or had reported an unusual odor.

"Mass psychogenic illness," as these incidents are sometimes called, aren't merely dismissed by public health experts. For one thing, the patients are not faking their symptoms; they do indeed feel sick. Then there is the disruption to the school or other institution where the incident occurs. But perhaps the feature of greatest concern is the similarity that psychogenic events share with bioterror scenarios. In the hours or days it takes to investigate such an incident, the school, or community, or even the nation, may be tossed by waves of fear.

---

Looking at, touching, listening to, and sometimes smelling patients provides doctors with clues that, in combination with medical histories, provide a reasonable diagnosis in most cases. Nevertheless, with the explosion in medical technology, will physicians continue to rely on their sense and direct contact with patients?

Many young physicians will recount the arduous process they went through learning to do physical exams as students . . . and then point out that in practice they zip through exams, while devoting more and more hours to interpreting test results. Many physicians have mixed feelings about the trend; recognizing the power of modern tests, while clinging to the personal connection between doctor and patient that the physical examination represents and fosters.

But when it comes to the odd cases that no amount of listening and palpating can resolve, there is no hesitation about engaging testing technology. Certainly that's how medicine is practiced in the world of *House, M.D.* Indeed, Dr. House and the team would be spending far too much time sitting at the table by the whiteboard tossing hypotheses into the air if they didn't have some tests to order. So let's head to the lab.

# THREE

# Let's Run Some Tests

**D**r. House relies heavily on a penetrating sense of human nature to reach his diagnoses. He uses his experience and understanding of patients to reveal the maladies they are most likely to be suffering. But there's nothing like a tox screen or MRI to start settling key questions.

## Lab Tests

Most medical decision-making, and certainly every life-threatening and complex case of the sort seen on *House, M.D.*, involves laboratory testing. Samples of blood, urine, spinal fluid, organ tissue, and even bits of DNA are able to reveal more and more about what is happening inside a patient's body.

"So much more is involved than just physical examination, which obviously was more important in eras gone by," says Fred H. Rodriguez, Jr., M.D. Dr. Rodriguez teaches courses on laboratory medicine at the Louisiana School of Medicine in New Orleans and he was the 2005–2006 president of the American Society for Clinical Pathology.

Dr. House and his colleagues perform a barrage of tests on most of their patients, yet they must be selective. Ordering too many tests can be as bad as or worse than not ordering enough. The flood of results would probably drown the important information and carry the doctors away in the wrong direction.

As one review of the evidence supporting laboratory tests put it: "One of the key deficiencies in the scientific literature on diagnostic tests often is the absence of an explicit statement of the clinical need, i.e., the clinical or operational question that the use of the test is seeking to answer." In other words, all too often tests are ordered without a clear understanding of how the results will be used. It is a commonly believed myth that more information is always better or that somehow test results will reveal important answers. In reality, asking the right questions is the most important part of the process, followed by using only those tests that are likely to answer those questions.

"No one says, 'Here's a blood specimen. Do all the tests you can do and send me the results.' The amount of data that the requesting physician would have to process would be just overwhelming," Dr. Rodriguez says. "So there is a selection process based on training and experience."

While it may be natural to think that more information is a good thing when trying to find out what's wrong with a patient, experts say that's often not true. Tests come with costs, financial and otherwise. In "Paternity" (1-02), Cuddy berates House for ordering a $3,200 DNA test in order to settle a bet. Most medical tests are not that expensive, but the totals can add up quickly and insurance may or may not cover the bill. Of course, even when insurance does pay for testing, health plans and public agencies just factor those costs into premiums and taxes. Often though, the immediate costs of medical testing to patients can be measured in terms of anxiety and follow-up procedures. These costs have to be balanced against the potential benefits of the information.

"When you are ordering a test, after taking a history and examining the patient, based on that body of knowledge, that information should guide you in your selection of tests. Before ordering a test, you should have a hypothesis. 'I'm going to predict that by doing this test, this is the answer I'm going to get, and it's going to confirm,' or 'I'm ordering the test because I'm expecting it to be negative and it will exclude something for me. And then based on the data I'll be able to narrow down the possibilities,'" Dr. Rodriguez says. "The attitude of: 'Well, I don't know what this test is going to show, but I'm going to order it and once it gets back it's going to tell me what I need to know,' that attitude is dealing with the situation from a position of grave weakness, rather than trying to select your test processes from a position of strength."

One of the more controversial tests developed in recent years can determine whether or not a woman carries BRCA1, the so-called breast cancer gene. As with most tests, the BRCA1 test does not offer a yes or no answer about whether a woman will get breast cancer. A positive test indicates that a woman has a higher than average risk of developing breast cancer. How much higher is also a matter of scientific debate.

But the real question for a woman contemplating breast cancer gene testing (or anyone thinking about any test) is, "What will I do with the result?" Some women who tested positive for the BRCA1 gene mutation have chosen to have mastectomies even though they don't have any detectable cancer. Other women choose to keep their breasts, but get frequent mammograms and clinical breast examinations.

On the flip side, a negative test does not mean a woman won't ever get breast cancer, just that her risk may be closer to average.

The situation is different, of course, for a patient in the hospital who is clearly sick . . . and where laboratory testing may help doctors figure out what is wrong. But when the results come back from the lab, doctors have to decide which results are relevant. The report will state whether the results are within a normal range, which raises the question: what's normal?

In the episode "Spin" (2-06), a professional bicycle racer collapses. His blood test results appear normal, but Chase wonders if what is normal for most people is out of whack for this patient. Perhaps his "normal" results actually could be showing white cell counts that are elevated for this patient, thus suggesting an infection.

Normal does not mean the same thing as healthy. We don't understand enough about the human body to be able to calculate some objective list of all the "healthiest" values of different substances. For the most part, the values we get on test reports are based on measurements taken from large groups of people who seem to be healthy; at least those who don't have any known symptoms or history of disease. Like many things in nature, the results gathered from these survey participants produce a bell-shaped curve on a graph, the so-called normal distribution, meaning that a lot of people had results somewhere in the middle, but a few people had results that are substantially higher or lower, even though they appeared to be healthy at the time of the test.

It is general practice to trim off the "tails" of the bell curve and then define a normal range for those test results that will include about nine out of ten people in the survey. For example, the range for a total white blood cell count is often put at between 4,000 and 10,000 cells per cubic millimeter of blood. In other words, two perfectly healthy people can have white blood cell counts that are very different. Indeed, one could have a count more than twice as high as the other and still be considered within the normal range.

People who are clearly sick don't all have the same numbers on a specific test. Their results range just like those of healthy people. And that range for people with a disease often overlaps with the range of results from healthy people.

Sometimes other factors are involved. For instance, cholesterol levels are increasingly compared against desired levels, rather than the average levels. So when your doctor says your cholesterol is a bit high, it may be perfectly normal, even though it indicates that you have a higher risk of heart disease than people with lower cholesterol levels.

Although people, even physicians, often refer to normal or abnormal test results, the official term for the values on a test report is the reference range. The term is meant to highlight the fact that the results are just meant to help compare an individual patient to the population in general, not to declare what's normal or healthy.

There is no clear cutoff between normal and abnormal for most clinical measurements and laboratory tests. Since normal limits for many laboratory tests are established by statistical methods, it is imperative that the clinician base his interpretation of the laboratory results on the clinical situation. In addition, a clinician should realize that the prevalence of disease is affected by the setting in which he practices, and the manner in which he uses a clinical test can affect the predictive value of the test used.

—From W.B. Applegate, "Decision Theory for Clinicians: Uses and Misuses of Clinical Tests," *Southern Medical Journal*, April 1981, p. 468

Once again, the lesson is that physicians have to look at the whole patient and decide where test results fit into a complete picture. Cases where a single number determines the outcome are the exception, rather than the rule.

In several episodes of *House, M.D.*, test results were not what they seemed at first. Sometimes, as in "Spin," drugs that the patient had been taking secretly to boost his athletic performance masked an underlying disease. In other cases, the patient's diet affected what the tests showed. In "The Socratic Method" (1-06), the patient was having problems with bleeding and clotting at the same time, even though the tests for clotting time appeared normal. Her monotonous diet of hamburgers had caused a vitamin K deficiency, which led to her blood problems, while fooling the standard test.

Doctors have to be careful not to be misled by test results when treating patients with anticlotting drugs, such as warfarin, that are meant to reduce the risk of a heart attack, stroke, or other clot-related threats. A patient who loves collard greens or other leafy, green vegetables may need a higher dose of the drugs to get the desired effect. But when fresh greens go out of season and the patient's diet changes, the drug dose that was correctly balanced in the summer may be too high, leading to potentially dangerous bleeding.

## Who's in the Lab?

On *House, M.D.*, Chase, Cameron, or Foreman are often seen working in the lab, looking at tissue samples or waiting for a machine to finish processing a chemical analysis.

"That is fiction," Dr. Rodriguez says. Performing laboratory tests not only requires special expertise, it is tightly regulated by federal and state laws. "A doctor at the bedside would not be permitted to do most tests."

CLIA, the Clinical Laboratory Improvement Amendments of 1988, is a federal law that sets standards for all medical laboratories, from those in the best-equipped academic medical centers down to closet-sized labs in doctors' offices. The main impetus for this stricter regulation was an investigation by the *Wall Street Journal* newspaper in 1987. The series of articles revealed a variety of sloppy or even fraudulent practices, including labs that pushed their employees to process four times as many Pap smear specimens as experts recommended. Pap smears can reveal early signs of cervical cancer. The health and lives of many women were put at risk, both because some lethal cancers were not detected, but also because other women underwent further testing or procedures prompted by positive reports that were wrong.

"Any test that's going to make a difference in how you are going to take care of a patient is covered by this law," Dr. Rodriguez says. "Not that doctors can't do their own tests, but they would have to be assessed at least once a year to the satisfaction of reviewers."

A physician who specializes in laboratory tests and the study of the body's fluids and tissues is a pathologist. Lab tests are also performed by technicians and others trained and licensed to perform the tests, but it is a physician who interprets what the results mean for patients. With over 2,000 different lab tests available, when a patient needs specialized testing, it is a pathologist who typically helps the attending physician select the tests that are most likely to provide useful answers . . . and then the pathologist often consults with the attending physician when the results are known.

The lag between ordering a medical test and getting back the results is much longer than it appears on TV. In the real world, complex tests, such as some genetic analyses, can take weeks.

Frequently used tests:

## "SED" RATE

One of the most frequently mentioned lab tests on *House, M.D.* is the "sed rate." The full name of the test is the erythrocyte sedimentation rate. It may be identified by its initials: ESR. The ESR test was introduced in 1921. It is a measure of how fast erythrocytes, red blood cells, settle in uncoagulated blood. The rate at which the cells drop is influenced by the amount of fibrinogen in the blood.

The ESR test can indicate the presence of inflammation, which can suggest that the patient is fighting an infection, cancer or perhaps arthritis, vascular diseases, or other conditions.

As a broad screening test, the ESR does not provide proof of a specific condition. It merely indicates whether the patient's blood appears to be normal or whether something may be amiss.

## CHEM-7

CHEM-7 is another test commonly ordered by House and his team.

The test is really seven different tests that look at the chemistry of a sample of blood serum, the part of blood without red, white, or other cells. The CHEM-7 report shows the levels of BUN (blood urea nitrogen), chloride, carbon dioxide, creatinine, glucose, potassium, and sodium in the patient's blood serum.

This sort of test is also called a basic metabolic panel, although the BMP typically includes a measurement of calcium, making eight tests in all.

## CBC

While the CHEM-7 looks at seven aspects of blood serum, the CBC takes a broader view of the red cells, white cells, and platelets. CBC stands for complete blood count. It includes measurements of hemoglobin, the protein in red blood cells that carries oxygen. Many diseases affect the levels of blood cells and other factors measured by the CBC, making it a good starting point for a diagnostic investigation.

Elevated white blood cell counts may indicate an infection or some types of cancer, such as leukemia. Paradoxically, a decreased white blood count may also be a sign of a severe infection. High red blood cell counts can be a sign of severe diarrhea or dehydration.

Low red blood cells can indicate anemia. High platelet counts may indicate a risk the patient's blood could form dangerous clots. Low platelets may indicate a risk of bleeding.

CBC tests used to be ordered as part of almost all routine exams. They are used more sparingly now, but they are still a common part of the broad search at the beginning of the diagnostic process.

## "TOX" SCREEN

A newsletter from the Yale-New Haven Hospital in Connecticut called the "tox" screens "probably the most misunderstood tests performed by the Clinical Lab." Although the tox screen is referred to on *House, M.D.* as though it were a single test, toxicology screens actually describe a variety of tests used to look for toxins, including drugs, in urine, blood, and other body fluids and tissues. The newsletter article pointed out that tox screens cannot rule out every type of poisoning or exposure to every possible substance. There are just too many possibilities.

When physicians order a tox screen, they actually are requesting one of a variety of specific testing procedures. So before the test is ordered, the physician must decide what she thinks might be causing a patient's problem, based on the history or other information.

One of the most common tox screens involves thin-layer chromatography (TLC) on an extract of urine. Levels of substances that are in the body may be concentrated in the urine. A positive test indicates exposure, but other tests are needed to determine how much of a substance is in the body and when the exposure occurred. Sometimes this sort of testing identifies metabolites, or breakdown products, of a substance that may linger in the body longer.

Blood samples are typically analyzed with gas chromatography or specific tests meant to detect individual substances, such as street drugs that may cause a dangerous overdose.

On *House, M.D.*, the doctors frequently remark that a patient's tox screen was "clean" or negative. However, that fact does not prove conclusively that the patient was not exposed to anything, since tox screens detect only the specific substances being tested for (perhaps a few dozen in many hospital laboratories) and then only when the levels are above a certain threshold. A negative tox screen just reduces the likelihood the patient was exposed to the substance that the doctor was suspicious of.

In the episode "Poison" (1-08), the tox screen on a patient was negative, but Chase pointed out that the result could just mean that the boy was exposed to something they had not tested for. Indeed, it was ultimately determined that pesticide poisoning was the cause of the patient's illness, but it was not a substance that would have been flagged by the tox screens that were first ordered.

In addition to identifying drugs in possible overdose situations, tox screens are used in a wide variety of situations, including suspected workplace exposures to toxic materials, household poisonings, and also as part of the examination of people who show signs of depression, bipolar disorder, and other psychiatric issues, in order to make sure that drug use does not explain the symptoms. Tox screens may also be used before declaring a patient brain dead; again, just to make sure that a drug is not suppressing brain wave activity.

## GENETIC TESTS

There is an expanding galaxy of tests that look at DNA and other genetic material, far too many to begin to discuss here. The uses of genetic tests are both similar to, and yet very different from, those of other tests. Like many blood tests, DNA tests can be used to identify the source of a patient's symptoms. In "Daddy's Boy" (2-05), the team performed a DNA test for type 2 neurofibromatosis, a type of tumor that can grow on nerves.

But unlike most blood tests, rather than just measure what is currently going on inside a patient's body, many genetic tests can predict the risk of developing certain problems. The BRCA1 breast cancer gene test discussed earlier is one example of a test that predicts risk, rather than identifying disease. A test that offers an even starker prediction is the test for Huntington's Disease. A positive test result for this inherited disorder means almost certain early death, preceded by several years of declining mental and physical function. Children of those with Huntington's Disease could be tested. But most experts and advisory groups say testing should wait until the children grow up and can decide as adults whether they want to know their likely fate, since there is no treatment or other action known to delay or prevent the onset of symptoms.

Other tests with a genetic component may be recommended for children, because treatment or preventive action can make a difference. Almost all newborns in the United States are screened for phenylketonuria (PKU), an inherited disorder that can lead to retardation and other problems if not recognized shortly after birth. When it is identified early, a careful diet can effectively protect the health of the child. Because screening and treatment are so effective, PKU testing of newborns is required in every state.

One of the most important and challenging features of many tests for inherited disorders is that they do not provide results only for the individual, but in essence test a whole family. If one person in a family is tested for breast cancer genes or Huntington's or cystic fibrosis, the answers they get may reveal information about the risks faced by their relatives. Although individuals usually have a right to keep their medical test information confidential, genetic counselors will consult with people getting certain genetic tests, to discuss whether and how to inform other family members about results that may affect them, too.

Another kind of family consequence of genetic tests was illustrated in "Paternity" (1-02). DNA testing ordered by Dr. House revealed that the patient, a sixteen-year-old boy, was adopted. In this case, the parents knew their son wasn't their biological offspring. However, genetic counselors say it is not uncommon for their tests to reveal family secrets, including affairs. One family was puzzled when a middle-aged father began showing symptoms of Huntington's Disease. None of his direct ancestors had developed the disease. Then it became clear that his mother had had a secret affair with a family friend. Grandfather was not grandfather, after all. Such news of "misattributed paternity" can be understandably traumatic for a family. Genetic counselors struggle with how to warn people about the potential for genetic tests to uncover things that people might prefer remain hidden.

## Television Time Warp

The physicians on *House, M.D.* rarely wait long for test results. They request a test and the results are usually back by the next scene. Real-world testing usually takes longer, sometimes much, much longer.

While certain urgent tests can be performed in minutes, results typically are not sent back to the physician until hours or even days later . . . or maybe even weeks later. In the episode "Hunting" (2-07), Cameron requested a Kveim-Siltzbach test for sarcoidosis, which is a type of inflammation that produces small lumps of cells in various organs.

The test involves injecting a preparation made from a confirmed case of sarcoidosis under the skin of a patient, somewhat like a tuberculosis skin test, in order to see how the patient's body reacts. If a papule, a small bump, appears, then the test is positive and the patient probably has sarcoidosis. On *House, M.D.*, the Kveim-Siltzbach test results were back within a day. In reality the reaction takes a month or longer, which is one reason the test is rarely used.

Blood tells many tales. That's why it is so often tested. But there's also another reason: Getting blood for a test is relatively easy and safe. Of course, many people are squeamish about drawing blood and may draw only a thin line between phlebotomists and vampires . . . but in order to get an accurate diagnosis, or simply as part of a regular checkup, physicians routinely ask patients to open a vein.

Sometimes though, the answer isn't found in a blood sample . . . and a piece of some other tissue is required. Removing a tissue sample for diagnostic purposes is called a biopsy.

## Biopsies

Of all the biopsies depicted on *House, M.D.*, probably none triggers a stronger viewer reaction than the retinal biopsy performed in the second episode, "Paternity." The patient's brain might be under attack by a mutant measles virus. Rather than biopsy the brain itself, the team opts to push a big needle through the eye to get at the retina on the rear wall. Foreman points out that although the needle looks scary, the patient's eye has been paralyzed, he won't feel a thing, and the eye won't be damaged.

---

### Mutant Measles

Beyond the imposing retinal biopsy diagnostic procedure, the "Paternity" episode shows an uncommon, but quite real, form of measles that can lurk for years or decades before attacking the brain.

Measles is one of the most infectious viruses known. Although only thirty-seven cases were reported in the United States in 2004, a new record low, before measles vaccination it was a common childhood disease. In most cases, measles symptoms last about a week, causing rash, fever, cough, runny nose, and red, watery eyes. It is still common in parts of the world without routine vaccination. Although it is fatal in less than 1 percent of cases, measles kills almost a million children in the world every year.

But the typical, brief measles illness may not be the end of the viral threat. Sometimes the measles virus goes into hiding, emerging years or even decades later as a deadly brain disease known as subacute sclerosing panencephalitis (SSPE). Because of measles vaccination, SSPE has almost disappeared in the United States. By 1980, the rate of SSPE had dropped to about one case per year for every 17 million people.

In "Paternity," a teenage boy adopted just after birth developed double vision and night terrors. House noticed a myoclonic jerk: twitching of the boy's legs that usually happens only when people are falling asleep. Each of these symptoms is a sign of SSPE, but also of other, more common health problems. Eventually, House learns that the boy's birth mother had not been vaccinated against measles, which left her son vulnerable during his first few months of life, when he should have been protected by maternal antibodies.

There have been case reports of SSPE in the children of mothers who were not vaccinated, even though the patients had received measles shots and had not shown signs of typical measles infections in childhood. Presumably the virus can be dormant for many years. In one study, the oldest patient developed SSPE at age twenty-six, almost twenty-four years after having childhood measles.

Vision problems may precede other neurological symptoms by several years.

"I have a case of an Australian girl who presented at age twenty-five with school deterioration, some memory difficulties, and attention/concentration problems. These signs are usually missed because they seem so nonspecific. She had a chorioretinitis (an inflammation of blood vessels in the retina of the eye) diagnosed by an ophthalmologist at age nine, but it was dismissed as some kind of nonspecific, perhaps viral, infection," says Generoso G. Gascon, M.D., who is professor emeritus, Clinical Neuroscience and Pediatrics, at Brown University School of Medicine in Providence, Rhode Island.

Dr. Gascon says that by the time myoclonic spasms appear, the patient is already in the second stage of SSPE.

SSPE usually leads to convulsions, dementia, coma, and death. Injecting interferon, a protein that spurs the immune system into action, directly into the brain is one of the treatment options for SSPE. Oral isoprinosine, also called inosiplex, is also one of the first treatment options. In one study, about a third of patients stabilized or improved after six months with either isoprinosine alone or in combination with alpha interferon injected into the ventricles of the brain. Antiviral drugs, such as ribavirin, also have been tried in SSPE patients. Other studies indicate that about 5 to 10 percent of SSPE patients recover on their own.

Patients also receive drugs, such as the antiepileptic drug carbamazepine, to manage the muscle spasms caused by SSPE.

At the end of "Paternity," the teenage patient is shown playing lacrosse once again, apparently cured. In reality, long-term survival is unusual. Most SSPE patients steadily decline and die, no matter what treatment is given.

Nevertheless, Dr. Gascon says occasional success stories motivate him and other experts in SSPE.

"I've had perhaps four or five patients over the last twenty-five to thirty years, who've had that kind of recovery, and I know there are sporadic patients around the world like that," Dr. Gascon says. "It's those kinds of results that keep those of us who are interested in SSPE continuing to try to treat these patients."

Few biopsies are as dramatic as a needle through the eye. Biopsies are performed routinely to follow up the findings of mammograms, prostate cancer tests, and more.

Stereotactic needle biopsy is a popular way to find out whether a lump seen on a mammogram is a tumor or merely a cyst. Before the technique was introduced, many women underwent minor surgical procedures, so that physicians could remove and inspect the suspicious lump. As an alternative to surgically removing the lump, when the lump can be felt, a physician can simply insert a needle and draw out some cells. A pathologist then examines the cells for signs of cancer.

Stereotactic needle biopsy takes the technique a step further, by allowing physicians to find lumps even when they cannot be felt. The woman lies face down on a special table with an opening for her breast. A special type of mammography device takes images of the breast from multiple angles, and then a computer calculates the precise location of the suspicious lump. What's more, the computer then controls a biopsy needle mounted beneath the table, guiding it directly to the lump. That way the doctor knows that the cells being examined are from the same spot that looked suspicious on the mammogram.

Men also get their share of needle biopsies—for prostate cancer. When a blood test or prostate exam raises concern about cancer, samples of the prostate can be retrieved by needle biopsy. In most cases the physician performing the biopsy is guided by ultrasound. The technique is not as precise as stereotactic needle biopsy of the breast, however. Even when several samples are retrieved, small tumors may be missed.

Biopsies are not always performed with needles. The term simply refers to retrieving some tissue for examination by whatever method is appropriate. Some biopsies are minor surgical procedures. A biopsy of the lungs may be performed with a bronchoscope.

A bronchoscope is a device with a flexible tube that can be inserted down the throat and into the lungs. With fiber optics, the physician can see where the end of the tube is going. She can suck fluids up a tube for examination. The doctor can collect solid tissue by using tiny forceps inserted down the tubing.

Samples from biopsy procedures, whatever the technique, are sent to a pathology lab for examination under a microscope or analysis by other methods.

## Imaging

In almost every episode, the team gets imaging scans of patients. Most often the scans are MRIs or CTs, but they also sometimes use ultrasound or nuclear medicine scans. Each of these technologies has strengths and weakness and each is used in specific ways to help physicians make a diagnosis or guide treatment.

### MRI

MRI stands for magnetic resonance imaging, also called NMR or nuclear magnetic resonance.

Powerful magnets cause hydrogen atoms in the body, which are part of water and other molecules, to line up along the field direction. Radio frequency pulses then cause some of the hydrogen atoms to move and emit energy. The energy is detected and mapped by a computer to produce the MRI scan that a radiologist interprets.

MRI scans are typically used to view soft tissues, anything from the brain to the abdomen to muscles and tendons.

The original name for the technique, nuclear magnetic resonance, fell out of use in part because of concerns that people might think that the devices or the scanning energy were radioactive. They aren't. In this case, the word nuclear simply refers to the nucleus of the atoms that are affected by the magnetic fields and radio frequency pulses.

There are also newer types of MRI machines called functional MRIs. Instead of taking still pictures of the body's interior, functional MRIs (sometimes called f-MRIs) can make movies. The f-MRIs are used in brain research. As study participants perform various tasks, the scan can show which parts of the brain are being used.

## CT

CT stands for computed tomography, also called a CAT scan, short for computed axial tomography.

The name refers to the use of computers to create two-dimensional or even three-dimensional images from a series of X-ray readings. The device emits a narrow X-ray beam that is measured by a detector on the other side of the patient being scanned. The intensity of this beam reveals how much of the X-ray energy was absorbed or scattered as the beam passed through. That single bit of information does not reveal very much, but with a computer running a series of complex calculations, all the little bits of information from beams sent through the body at all angles can be merged together to produce a detailed image of the interior of the patient.

CT images of soft tissues are generally less detailed than those produced by MRIs. A standard CT image does not show blood vessels very well. However, if a so-called contrast solution is injected into the blood stream, then a CT image can produce a valuable view of blood flow and abnormalities in blood vessel structure. The contrast solution strongly absorbs X-rays, so that the blood vessels stand out brightly on the CT images.

CT scanners are designed to use the minimum necessary amount of X-ray radiation. The risk of cancer or other radiation-related problems from a single scan is extremely low. However, the risk does rise if a patient needs multiple scans or ongoing monitoring. In addition, doctors would rarely do a CT scan of the belly of a pregnant woman. Particularly in the first few weeks of pregnancy, the radiation could raise the risk of malformations or cancer in the fetus.

## X-RAY

The term commonly means using X-rays to get a single two-dimensional image of bones and major features in the body. The radiation is similar to that used in CT scanning, but there's no computer manipulation of the data to create different views. X-rays are the oldest form of medical imaging. In 1895, German physicist Wilhelm Conrad Roentgen discovered how to produce high-energy radiation that passed through many solid objects the way normal light passes through translucent glass. This "X" radiation affected photographic film and so the technique could be used to produce shadowy images of the internal structure of the body.

Modern machines produce far sharper images, of course, and they use much less radiation. X-rays are routinely used to check teeth for cavities, diagnose broken bones, look for tuberculosis infections in the lungs, and more. At one time, X-rays were part of routine checkups, but that practice faded a generation ago amid concerns about unnecessary exposure to radiation. Similarly, early hopes that regular chest X-rays could help detect the early signs of lung cancer in smokers dwindled as studies showed that by the time lung tumors became detectable, they were usually too far along to be treated successfully. There are now studies underway to see if the latest high-resolution CT scanners are useful for smokers.

Specialized applications of X-rays include angiography, mammography, and bone density tests.

Angiography uses contrast fluids injected into arteries to help produce detailed images of blood flow. The technique can find and measure narrowings or blockages that can cause heart attacks or strokes. The images can be done in real time, to help guide physicians using catheters or other methods to restore blood flow. Angioplasty and cardiac stents are frontline therapies for heart attacks and chest pain due to blood flow problems using catheters. Unlike most heart bypass operations, the patient's chest remains closed, so these treatments rely on angiography to show cardiologists the location of the tips of the catheters they are using.

Mammography is the use of an X-ray machine that is specifically designed to look for tumors and other abnormalities in the breast.

Bone density scans, which are used to check for signs of osteoporosis, use X-rays, but not to create a conventional image. The important information here is how strong the bones are. By passing X-rays through the body, the scanner can calculate how dense the bones are by how much of the X-ray energy was blocked

Although the key difference between standard X-rays and CT scans is that CT scanners use computer calculations to create the image, standard X-rays are going digital. Increasingly, special digital camera-like devices are replacing film. Computers are also being used to enhance and even start examining all types of images, including standard X-rays.

## NUCLEAR MEDICINE

Rather than send a beam of energy through the body to reveal what's inside, nuclear medicine generally uses slightly radioactive fluids that are either infused into or ingested by the patient in order to find tumors, tiny bone fractures, or other abnormalities. The radioactive substance, called a tracer, is formulated to collect at an area of interest or attach itself to a tumor or other abnormality. A camera that can detect the low-level radiation sees the buildup of the tracer as a hot spot.

The images are usually rather fuzzy, not showing details of the internal structures of the body. But standard X-rays and most other imaging techniques have to be aimed at a specific area of the body. That means doctors need to have some idea where to look. One advantage of nuclear medicine tracers is that they can help find tumors when doctors don't know where to look. For instance, in patients who have symptoms suggesting cancer may be somewhere in the body, a nuclear medicine scan may reveal the tumor's hiding spot. The tracers are also used to monitor some cancer patients for recurrences after they've been treated, since they may be able to locate microscopic tumors.

PET scans (positron-emission tomography) are one application of nuclear medicine. A PET scan has some similarity with CT scans. A ring of detectors picks up low-level radioactive emissions and then a computer uses tomography to assemble the data into an image. The difference is that during a PET scan the radiation comes from a tracer substance introduced into the patient's body, whereas CT scans involve X-rays that come from an external emitter and pass through the patient's body before hitting the detector.

PET scans are often used to look for cancer, because tumor cells tend to consume more glucose than most normal cells; so a radioactive tracer made with glucose will concentrate in the tumor, thus producing a bright area on the PET image. PET scans are also used by clinicians and researchers to study brain activity. When a region of the brain is active it uses more glucose, so it gets brighter on a PET scan using a glucose tracer. For example, PET scans have helped researchers identify what parts of the brain are involved in sight and other senses, where memories are stored, and which areas are stimulated when a smoker sucks on a cigarette.

SPECT (Single photon emission computed tomography) works much like PET scanning, but the tracer is designed to give off a different type of radiation. SPECT images are less detailed than PET scans, but the devices are less expensive and more widely available.

## ULTRASOUND

Ultrasound imaging devices are becoming so common in medical practice that they threaten the role of the venerable stethoscope as a physician's first tool to glimpse inside a patient's body. As the name indicates, the devices use high-frequency sound waves, like sonar, to create an image. Unlike X-ray beams that go through the patient to a detector, ultrasound energy bounces back to the transducer, which both emits and then picks up the sound waves, hence ultrasound's nickname: "echo."

Ultrasound does not raise the type of safety concerns X-rays do; nor are the machines nearly as costly as MRIs. Indeed, ultrasound machines continue to shrink both in terms of cost and size. There are handheld devices that cost less than $1,000 that are meant to replace stethoscopes in certain situations.

Ultrasound is not only used to view fetuses and organs, it is particularly well suited to measuring blood flow, thanks to the Doppler effect. The Doppler effect is what you hear when the siren of a speeding ambulance or police car sounds higher pitched when it is racing toward you and then drops in pitch as it passes. This change in pitch can be used to calculate the speed at which blood is flowing toward or away from the ultrasound transducer. Doppler ultrasound is often used to detect problems with heart valves by sensing when blood is squirting through a valve that should be tightly shut.

Elliot Fishman, M.D., at Johns Hopkins University, routinely sees the type of tough cases that might find their way to Dr. House, cases that have stumped other doctors.

He recalls a patient he saw recently.

"The patient had a lot of vague symptoms—weight loss, wasn't feeling well. A lot of the blood values were off, the sedimentation rate was elevated. These were things that suggested a chronic process. Then we did a CT. There was a thought that maybe the patient had a malignancy somewhere. What we ended up finding was that the patient had a vasculitis; something called Takayasu's Arteritis, with a lot of thickening of vessel walls. It's treated with steroids. That's not a cure, but usually you can control it," Dr. Fishman says. "It was totally unexpected. No one had thought of it. But based on the CT it became very clear."

He says *House, M.D.* generally paints a realistic picture of doctors using medical imaging to help solve complex cases . . . and to identify the rare conditions that do indeed pop up.

"With scans, you can really see what's in there," Dr. Fishman says.

CTs and MRIs can actually see too much, prompting anxiety and then further testing to check out apparent abnormalities that, in the end, do not present any health threat.

Researchers in Southern California reviewed more than a thousand whole-body CT scans performed at a for-profit scanning facility. Three out of four people who were scanned had decided on their own to get the test; in other words, they were not referred by a physician and so there was probably no clear medical issue that required an imaging test.

Almost all the scans, nine out of ten, found something, but that doesn't mean the scans prevented these people from getting sick or dying. In most cases, nothing was done, because the abnormality seen on the scans did not appear to be important. In about a third of the cases, the individuals were referred for further testing or other follow-up work.

Just imagine if everyone got a whole-body scan, just to see what's going on inside? The result would be millions of people getting further tests. And only rarely would something be discovered that was actually life threatening. What's more, even if something dangerous was found through such a test, it might not be treatable; so the ultimate fate of the patient would not change. The only thing the scan would do in such a case is give the patient the bad news earlier and probably increase the amount of testing, worry, and expense.

When individuals decide to get a screening scan without a doctor's referral, they usually pay out of pocket. A scan of the chest, abdomen, and pelvis in a mobile CT scanner can be had for $398. At the other end of the scale, a Hawaiian resort spa and scanning center offers airport pickup, lei greeting, spa treatments, meals, and two nights' lodging, in addition to five imaging tests and other exams, all for $4,000.

That hit to the wallet does dampen public enthusiasm for CT screening. According to a market survey performed by a medical imaging company in the Boston area, cost was the most common reason people cited for not wanting a CT scan. Recognizing that an initial test often raises new questions, this company includes a limited amount of follow-up testing in the basic package. "If somebody has something, particularly in the liver or the kidney, sometimes in the CT scan it looks like a cyst, but you just can't be one hundred percent sure, we will do an ultrasound to clarify that finding or the abnormality in the liver or the kidney, as part of the exam without charging extra for it. We are doing it so people leave with as few loose ends as possible," says Max Rosen, M.D. But he concedes scanning centers cannot offer a full workup after every scan that shows some sort of abnormality.

Radiologist James Borgstede, M.D., 2005–2006 Chair of the American College of Radiology Board of Chancellors, says the initial scans are not the problem. "The real problem is the false positives that come out of that screening scan. Who pays for those?" he asks. "You know, the patients will come in and pay the money for the scan, but then as soon as something is found in the scan, which is typically a false positive finding, then their insurance kicks in. And if you have a health care plan, now suddenly somebody in your plan gets one of these scans, that changes the profile of your health care plan and that, in effect, changes your premiums. So I think we have to think about this from an epidemiologic and a population basis."

Some experts go even farther, arguing that until CT screening proves its worth, individuals who opt for CT scans in the absence of symptoms or clear risk factors should bear the full cost of the consequences. Dr. Fishman, head of the Advanced Medical Imaging Laboratory at the Johns Hopkins Medical Institutions in Baltimore, Maryland, notes that a positive scan often leads to a steady stream of regular follow-up scans, a cash cow for scanners, but a drain on health plans. "As far as I'm concerned, they ought to do this: if you self-refer, you are responsible for everything," he argues. While he supports coverage of screening ordered by a physician as part of comprehensive care, Fishman warns about the cost to society of uncontrolled CT screening. "Truthfully, it could break the system. You start running up these costs chasing nonsensical things," he predicts. "I'm not here to have my insurance rates go up because people decide on their own they are going to go for studies at second-rate places and then get more studies to follow something that's of no importance."

The potential price tag for self-referred CT screening is as uncertain as potential health benefits. According to a published account of a plenary session debate on CT screening at the 2002 Scientific Assembly of the Radiological Society of North America (RSNA), Bruce Hillman, M.D., chair of Radiology at the University of Virginia in Charlottesville, said a study of CT scanning indicated that screening healthy fifty-year-old individuals for key cancers, aneurysms, and heart disease could cost $150,000 per year of life saved.[1] In other

1. RSNA 2002 meeting coverage by Diagnostic Imaging.com.

words, if you scanned a large group of fifty-year-old people who appeared to be healthy, you would probably discover some treatable cancers.

Say that twenty cancers were found and that each patient lived an average of five years longer because of the early detection and treatment. That would mean the screening program would get credit for a total of 100 years of extended life. According to Dr. Hillman's calculation, you would have to do $15 million dollars worth of screening to produce that result.

Other calculations produce lower cost estimates. In the RSNA debate, Michael Brant-Zawadzki, M.D., medical director of Radiology at Hoag Memorial Hospital in Newport Beach, California, pointed to other analyses of more limited screening for lung cancers that predict CT scanning might cost less than $50,000 per year of life saved.

While the use of scanning technology may be realistic, there's something very unreal about medical imaging on *House, M.D.*: radiologists are invisible. Chase, Foreman, or Cameron usually are at the control board and House even stops in on occasion to monitor things. That's not how scans are done in most hospitals.

Dr. Borgstede, a radiologist in Colorado Springs, says attending physicians rarely even look at the finished scans. That's the job of the radiologist.

"Few physicians actually come down to look at the pictures. Some of them do, but that's not typical. They are relying on a report. And even if they do come down to look at the films, the more sophisticated the imaging test, the more they rely on the radiologist for the interpretation," Dr. Borgstede says.

Dr. Fishman agrees, noting that radiologists are trained to recognize telltale patterns in images. He says that a radiologist in a referral center like his, who sees many scans from many complex cases, has the experience to recognize unusual patterns that may change a diagnosis.

For instance, a woman with symptoms of liver disease had undergone a scan before being referred to an oncologist at Johns Hopkins.

"The outside scan was read as liver metastasis," he says. That diagnosis typically has a grim prognosis. But then Dr. Fishman took a closer look.

"Ends up that what this woman had was hydatid disease, which is a very unusual infection of the liver. It's seen in South American countries, caused by a parasite found in sheep. This woman was from Washington, but it turns out she was from Peru and had probably had the parasite since she was a child," he says.

"She had been sent to Hopkins for resection of a hepatic tumor, rather than hydatid disease. As a tumor, it was unresectable, there were too many lesions. As hydatid disease, it was treatable."

---

## Sensitivity and Specificity

With any type of test, there is a balance between how sensitive it is and how specific it is.

Sensitivity is how often the test will detect the thing being tested for. So a test that has a sensitivity of 90 percent will give a positive result to ninety out of 100 people who actually have what you are looking for.

Specificity is how often a negative result is correct; that is, that someone who does not have the disease or condition gets the correct test result. A test that is 90 percent specific will give a negative result to ninety out of 100 people who are free of the thing being tested for.

In most cases, a test that is more sensitive will be less specific and vice versa. In other words, if you want to find every case possible, the trade-off is incorrectly identifying more people as possibly having something they don't really have. That outcome is called a false positive. When a test incorrectly says someone doesn't have the disease, when they actually do, the result is called a false negative.

Take mammograms as an example: The more detailed the scan and the more cautious the radiologist interpreting it, the higher the likelihood that something will be identified as suspicious, perhaps catching a tiny breast cancer. Of course, the more sensitive the testing, the more likely it will pick up a shadow that isn't really cancer. On the other hand, trying to be more specific, so that you don't unnecessarily worry women who don't have cancer, raises the risk of missing a small tumor.

Interpreting sensitivity and specificity can be tricky, in part because interpreting results does not depend only on the accuracy of the test but also on how common the condition is.

Consider this scenario: In a city of 1,000,000 people, there's a disease that affects one in 100 people. That means that there are probably 10,000 people in the city with the disease.

Imagine that you have a test for the disease that has a sensitivity of 99 percent and a specificity of 98 percent. Sounds pretty good, doesn't it? The test will probably identify 9,900 of the 10,000 people with the disease.

On the other hand, the 98 percent specificity means that out of every 100 healthy people tested, two will be told incorrectly that they may have the disease. Since 10,000 people have the disease, that means that the remaining 990,000 people in the city are healthy. In this case then, the 98 percent sensitivity means almost 20,000 people (2 percent of 990,000) will be told they tested positive for a disease they don't really have.

Of course, with a screening test neither patient nor doctor knows in advance if the patient has the disease. All they know is the test result. Looking at the numbers in this scenario again shows that all together there will be 29,700 positive test results (the 9,900 "true" positives plus the 19,800 "false" positives.) Since 9,900 out of the 29,700 positive test results are "true," there is a one in three chance that any individual positive test result is true. Or flipping it around, two out of three people told that they had a positive test result do not actually have the disease.

Now consider what happens with less common diseases. Say in that same city of 1,000,000 people, the disease you are testing for affects only one person in 1,000. That means that there are probably 1,000 people in the city with the disease.

A test with a sensitivity of 99 percent and a specificity of 98 percent would probably identify 990 of the 1,000 people with the disease.

But remember that the remaining 999,000 people in the city are healthy and 2 percent of those healthy people will be given a "false" positive test result.

Testing everyone in the city would produce about 20,970 positive test results (the 990 "true" positives plus 19,980 "false" positives.) Since only 990 out of the 20,970 positive test results are "true," the likelihood of any individual positive test result being true is less than 5 percent, meaning that nineteen times out of twenty a person with a positive test result will turn out to be healthy.

In many cases the thresholds for declaring a test "positive" or "negative" can be adjusted up or down by the way the test is made or how the results are interpreted. The threshold may be set rather low in cases where a disease has dire consequences and the follow-up to a screening test is relatively benign (maybe just a repeat of the first test, or another test that is somewhat more time consuming or costs a bit more, but doesn't carry any physical risk to the patient.) On the other hand, you might well want to set a higher threshold, and thus perhaps miss a few more cases, if the disease is not immediately dangerous or if the follow-up to a positive test is a surgical biopsy or other invasive procedure that you want to avoid, if possible.

Don't feel bad if the statistics confuse you. Sensitivity and specificity trip up many physicians, too. One survey found that only one out of five physicians correctly interpreted the meaning of a positive test result when they were given the test's sensitivity and specificity.

---

# MRI Safety

It's not surprising that almost all of the primary patients on *House, M.D.* get an MRI test at some point in the episode, since MRIs offer a unique and powerful method of probing deep into a patient's body.

They are increasingly popular in routine health care. There are now about 10,000 MRI machines in U.S. hospitals and clinics scanning about 10 million patients every year.

Safety rarely enters the discussion of whether or when to perform an MRI scan on a patient. That's mostly because MRI scans are indeed very safe. Unlike CT scanners, they don't use X-rays, nor do they involve radioactive tracers like PET scans or other forms of nuclear medicine, so there is not any concern about cancer risk or other effects of ionizing radiation.

It may seem that the only downside to MRIs is the cost, which can range from a few hundred dollars to well over a thousand dollars, depending on the area being scanned, the sophistication of the scanner, the extent of interpretation required, and the particular pricing policies of the institution that owns the scanner.

But nothing in life is totally without risk. Most metal must be kept clear of an MRI scanning room, because the extremely powerful magnets of the scanner can fling even very heavy objects at patients or anyone else in the room. An oxygen tank can become a deadly missile if left in the MRI room. Chairs, IV stands, floor buffers used by unwary cleaning staff, even shipping pallets have been sucked into MRI machines.

The other leading risk is damage to pacemakers, drug delivery pumps, and other devices implanted in patients. In "Histories" (1-10), Cuddy stopped an MRI scan just before the magnetic field was cranked up, because the patient had a surgical pin in her arm. She said that the magnet would have ripped the implant out of the patient's body. And a metal plate used to reconstruct a patient's jaw forced the team to figure out the cause of a stroke without the benefit of an MRI. However, in both these cases an MRI might still have been possible, because most orthopedic implants, such as replacement joints or screws to help heal broken bones, as well as most dental implants, are made out of nonmagnetic metals. Some implants often used in eye, brain, or blood vessel procedures may be magnetic and could be tugged by the MRI's magnetic field, with painful or possibly life-threatening consequences. Patients with any sort of implants need to alert their doctors and staff before an MRI scan, just to be safe.

According to reports filed with the FDA, there were about 300 safety incidents attributable to MRIs between 1995 and early 2005. Nine people died. One death was due to a flying object. Most of the deaths were due to the failure of an implanted pacemaker or other device.

The FDA statistics include only reported cases of actual harm. Close calls are not reported. A more comprehensive reporting system in Pennsylvania collected eighty-eight MRI-related incidents in the state in just sixteen months; a much higher rate of incidents than the FDA system records for the entire nation, although the Pennsylvania incidents were generally less serious than those reported to the FDA.

There are signs of improvements. Many newer implantable devices are less likely to be affected by magnetic fields. But the power of MRIs commands respect . . . and an alertness for items that might be flung or damaged by the scanners' extraordinary magnetic fields.

\* \* \*

## Let's Run Some Tests

High-tech medical technology offers information about what is happening inside patients that earlier generations of physicians could only dream of. But all that data comes with a new challenge: information overload. Which facts are critical and which are just irrelevant "noise"? Computers helped create the flood of data. They are also a vital part of efforts to make sense of it all.

# FOUR

# Is There a Computer in the House?

Could Dr. House ever be replaced by a computer? A machine would not display his gruff sarcasm, his disdain for authority, or his dependence on Vicodin. But could a computer match his flair for diagnosis?

"If you were to ask me, 'Do you know how to build a computer program that can outperform a very good clinician?' I would say, 'Yeah.'" That emphatic endorsement of machine ability comes from Professor Enrico Coiera, the director of the Centre for Health Informatics at the University of New South Wales in Sydney, Australia.

In one sense, every physician is already computer assisted. It is the only way for doctors to stay up-to-date.

A century ago, a good physician could reasonably stay abreast of the medical literature. Not today. Online medical search engines are essential to physicians researching cases that are either unusual or outside the usual flow of their practices. Medline, managed by the National Library of Medicine, contains about 13 million references to life sciences journal articles, mostly published in the last forty years. It also links many of those references to full-text digital copies of the articles.

Searches can be tailored to look at specific categories of clinical studies, but they can also look at different types of medical information. One growing category is that of "systematic reviews." These reports use sophisticated statistical methods to combine the results of multiple clinical trials in an attempt to get at the big picture; in other words, what is the state of the art, taking all the results from individual trials into account. The National Library of Medicine also has special search features that help find information on medical genetics, as well as health care quality and costs.

The pile of new journal articles keeps growing. In 2004, Medline added over 571,000 new references. That is more than twice the annual number of medical research articles produced in the early 1980s. Today's physicians are dealing with vastly more information than their predecessors. On average, a new medical citation is added to Medline every fifty-five seconds. Doctors cannot hope to keep up. They need help. Increasingly, that help comes from digital databases.

Professor Coiera points out that the leading online databases are not merely electronic versions of stacks of medical journals that the physician can browse. When someone enters search terms, the computer program seeks abstracts that contain relevant and up-to-date information. In essence, the computer is deciding what the physician should look at first.

PDAs, personal data assistants, such as Palm or Pocket PC handheld devices, are putting these databases in the coat pockets of more and more physicians. The PDAs usually also contain treatment guidelines, consensus statements, and checklists from public health agencies, medical societies, and the health care institutions the physicians work at.

The *Merck Manual*, considered the most widely used textbook in medicine, is an imposing leather-bound tome almost 3,000 pages long. But doctors can carry an electronic version in their PDAs. It's no featherweight. The PDA version of the *Merck Manual* contains enough information on conditions and symptoms that it could spoil the suspense of a number of episodes of *House, M.D.*

The case of a high school athlete who turned out to have a measles infection that was attacking his brain in "Paternity" (1-02) is an example. The hook that got Dr. House interested in the case was a myoclonic jerk, an involuntary muscle twitch. Most people experience them now and then as they are falling asleep, but Dr. House was intrigued when he saw the boy's leg twitch while he was wide awake.

If Dr. House or Foreman or Chase or Cameron had whipped out their PDAs and looked under "Myoclonus" in their electronic *Merck Manual*, they would have seen that the twitches occur normally when falling asleep and that hiccups are a common form of myoclonus affecting the diaphragm. But if they had scrolled down to less common conditions, they would have seen this listing: subacute sclerosing panencephalitis, a brain disorder caused by a latent measles infection, which is exactly what they eventually found.

As Professor Denis J. Protti wrote in an article for a British National Health Service web site, "As for PDA and other handheld and wireless devices, clinicians' use of these technologies is growing rapidly. Enabling ready access to multiple sources of patient information and medical knowledge in a variety of formats, intelligent mobile applications offer a sought after level of seamless efficiency for clinicians without disrupting patient-physician interactions. Providing the highest level of healthcare increasingly implies equipping clinicians in real-time with a breadth and depth of updated patient care information that was previously unattainable."

It is true that physicians memorize a vast amount of information about the human body and the ailments to which it is vulnerable. But gone are the days when a doctor's brain and office bookshelf held all the information needed. Especially when there is something unusual about a case, today's physicians reflexively turn to their handheld devices and computer screens for a cyber assist.

Computers are also doing real medical work in doctors' offices. For instance, most blood tests are interpreted by a machine.

"It's all behind the scenes. Patients don't know about it. You get your blood test back and you see something written down at the bottom saying you've got this disease or that disease and you think a human has done it; but more than likely it's been generated by a machine and then checked by a human," says Professor Coiera, who is the author of the *Guide to Health Informatics*.

At least three systems are commercially available that help radiologists to search mammograms for signs of breast cancer, although a human eye makes the final call. Computer-assisted detection is considered part of standard practice and insurers will pay for the use of the computer systems in certain applications, such as breast cancer detection.

Researchers are actively investigating other ways to use computers to pick out significant anomalies from the mountains of imaging data spewed out by increasingly sensitive MRI, CT, and PET and other types of scanning machines. Indeed, studies of whole-body scans find that they almost always detect some sort of anomaly, but the lumps are rarely dangerous. Sifting through all the high-resolution images to separate the things that might be important from all the background noise is a daunting task. Computers can help winnow the data.

Lung cancer is one focus of the work. Currently, lung cancer treatment rarely succeeds, in part because the cancer often has spread by the time the patient notices any symptoms. Newer CT scanners can find nodules in the lung when they are very small and relatively easy to surgically remove. However, many of these tiny lumps turn out not to be cancers, just as the majority of breast lumps turn out to be cysts or other masses that are probably not dangerous. So one challenge facing radiologists is deciding when a tiny spot on an image is worth investigating, and when it is better to leave it alone, thus sparing the patient from unnecessary invasive procedures.

There are a number of different artificial intelligence models that are used in medical applications. They each take a different path toward the goal of having a machine mimic some of the things people do when analyzing a problem.

Rule-based systems are one way to try to capture and computerize the thinking processes that people go through. In a way, computer programs that use a rule-based system are akin to familiar checklists that can guide a physician toward the correct diagnosis. For instance, when a patient comes in with fever and chills, there are a number of diseases that could be suspected. If the patient just returned from Africa, then malaria may move up near the top of the list of possible diagnoses. If not, then perhaps the problem may be a variety of viral pneumonia. This sort of IF>THEN process can be programmed into a computer.

These sorts of rule-based systems require explicitly describing the logical process that the programmers want to mimic, but they aren't the only way to computerize problem-solving.

Neural networks are based not on explicit checklists, but rather on a sort of model of the brain itself; that is, connections between neurons that are strengthened with use. Instead of inputting long lists of IF>THEN statements to guide the computer, a neural network is trained.

"You train the neural network on lots and lots of examples of what you want it to find, until it develops a sort of picture in its own mind of what it's looking for. Then the next time you show it an example, it decides either that looks like what you want or it doesn't look like it," Professor Coiera says.

Neural networks are well suited to reading electrocardiograms or scan images, tasks that involve recognizing patterns. However, Professor Coiera notes that while neural networks can connect a set of observations with a set of diagnoses, they aren't very good at explaining themselves.

"A neural net will never tell you why," he says.

And sometimes that explanation is vital, in order for the person reading the computer response to decide how much to rely on it.

Another type of computerized diagnostician may become more popular as more health records are themselves computerized. Probability networks are designed to take a look at a set of symptoms and other information and match them up with the most likely explanations. This type of system works better the more examples the computer has of real cases where a certain set of data described a certain disease. The growth of electronic health records will help provide probability network systems the depth of "experience" they need to make connections more accurately.

But how good could a computer be at picking out the right diagnosis when the condition is extremely rare or there is something odd about the symptoms . . . the kind of cases in which following all the usual procedures and common clues leads to the wrong conclusion?

"That's the money question. Computer systems are fantastic at the standard. That doesn't mean they won't pick up rare things, but they are going to be very good at doing things where they've got lots and lots of data. So if you've got a rare case that no one's ever seen before, because you've got two diseases and one is masking the other one, and such a case has hardly ever been seen, then the machine is not necessarily going to be very good at that," Professor Coiera says. "But you could still use the machine to find related cases."

Dr. House pulls rare cases out of his vast memory on a regular basis. For instance, in "Fidelity" (1-07) the team is searching for possible scenarios to explain how a woman who had never been out of the country could contract African sleeping sickness. The disease is typically spread by the tsetse fly. Dr. House says the patient could have been infected through sexual contact. He references a case report of sexual transmission of sleeping sickness that appeared in a Portuguese medical journal.

Of course, mortal physicians cannot keep up with the English-language medical literature, much less scan articles in every other tongue. But with a computer assist, they don't have to. Rather than relying on memory or personally searching the medical literature, physicians can use computers to speed up the process of casting a wide net for other cases that look like the patient being examined.

"That's an example of another type of system called case-based reasoning, where you can find cases very similar to the one you've just found: similar presenting symptoms and signs and data," Professor Coiera says.

Case-based reasoning may be the type of computer system that is actually the closest to mimicking how people actually think; that is, by incorporating all their experience, all the cases they treated, into the diagnostic process of the next case.

"It's all about prior exposure to similar cases, rather than capacity to reason about cases," Professor Coiera says.

"What we find is that it's the knowledge people have based on prior experience that is the most important feature that distinguishes them, as opposed to some sort of powerful generic reasoning skill. That flash of insight is probably actually a memory of a case they saw twenty years ago that was similar, or something they recollected from the medical literature," he says. "So it's not like they are just bringing things together. We think there is a strong case-based reasoning going on with these doctors where they are matching things with their past experience."

## Sleeping-Around Sickness

If Foreman, Chase, or Cameron had decided to check on Dr. House's obscure Portuguese reference, a computer search of the medical literature using the key words "sleeping sickness sexual transmission" would have led them to the January 17, 2004, issue of *The Lancet*. A letter, in English, not Portuguese, describes a case much like the one mentioned in the show.

The doctors wrote from Lisbon, Portugal, that they had treated a woman for African sleeping sickness, even though she had never traveled to Africa. They discovered that her partner, a Brazilian man who had been in Angola, was infected with trypanosome parasites, although he did not have any symptoms.

Sleeping sickness is usually transmitted through tsetse fly bites. Transmission through blood transfusions or contaminated needles also has been reported. But in this case, doctors believe the woman had been infected through sexual contact. Her nineteen-month-old son was also sick. Presumably, she passed on the parasites to him before birth.

In "Fidelity," House and his team were trying to determine whether their patient had sleeping sickness or tularemia, also known as "rabbit fever." Their diagnosis depended on whether the patient or her husband had had an affair, because extramarital sexual contact would make sleeping sickness more likely, based on the case report of sexual transmission in Portugal.

In the show, it was critical to make a correct diagnosis, because treatments for both diseases were thought to present serious, even life-threatening side effects. In reality, rabbit fever is usually treated with antibiotics, such as streptomycin, which are not unusually risky. One drug, chloramphenicol, may lead to aplastic anemia, a serious blood disorder, in some cases. However, chloramphenicol is rarely the first choice, though some experts report that it seems to do a better job than streptomycin of attacking the tularemia bacteria in cerebrospinal tissue.

The sleeping sickness drug depicted in this episode, melarsoprol, contains arsenic. It can be hazardous; more than one patient in twenty may die. Nevertheless, melarsoprol is routinely used in Africa to effectively treat sleeping sickness.

In the cases of the mother and son in Portugal, doctors reported that both were treated successfully with an alternate drug, eflornithine, which is considered to be less hazardous than melarsoprol.

---

In some ways, being a machine can be an advantage when it comes to making the correct medical diagnosis. Machines are not swayed by recent experience. If you flip a coin and get heads five times in a row, most people will bet on the next flip coming up tails; but a computer will correctly calculate that the odds are still fifty-fifty, regardless of the unusual streak.

In medicine, one of the difficult skills young doctors are expected to master is the ability to simultaneously look for common, run-of-the-mill diseases, while keeping their minds open to the possibility of weird rarities and refraining from prematurely fixing on any one diagnosis. Machines are unbiased and have no emotional attachment to a particular diagnosis.

Not surprisingly, people may be skeptical about machines encroaching on their territory. That sentiment is captured in the episode "Failure to Communicate" (2-10). As it turns out, the patient has malaria parasites in his brain, apparently the result of undergoing surgery in South America. Dr. House orders the team to visually check a blood sample, rather than processing it by computer. When Foreman sees the parasites under a microscope, he and Cameron blame the computer for missing the critical sign.

## Is There a Computer in the House?

But is it fair to blame the computer? The reason no one had suspected malaria earlier in the episode is that the patient had concealed the fact that he had been in South America, not even telling his wife. Malaria almost never appears in the United States, unless it is in a person who has traveled to a region where malaria is common. There was no reason to look for parasites until the patient's secret trip was uncovered.

---

Some of the computer systems available to physicians include the following:

**GIDEON** (Global Infectious Diseases and Epidemiology Network) is a commercially available computer system that is updated weekly with information on infectious disease outbreaks around the world. Users put in as much information as they have about the patient's symptoms and where the patient has been recently. Then the program lists possible diagnoses with probability rankings.

In a study done by GIDEON's developers, information on 495 patients was entered. The correct diagnosis was listed in almost 95 percent of the cases, and it was the first diagnosis listed in three out of four cases.

A demonstration example put together by the makers of the GIDEON system sounds very much like the kind of case that would find its way to Dr. House's door. A twenty-year-old man suddenly becomes ill after a trip to Thailand and Mongolia. At the hospital, his physician enters his symptoms, findings from the physical exam, and blood test results. At first, the software puts tuberculosis at the top of a list of several infectious diseases. If the ranking does not match the physician's expectations, she can ask for an explanation.

In this example, the physician then remembers that the patient mentioned rats entering his tent in Mongolia. Adding that piece to the history vaults plague to the top of the list, in part because the software is constantly updated, so it could factor in recent reports of plague in Mongolia.

The GIDEON software then provides details on the *Yersinia pestis* bacterium and recommended treatments. This type of decision support system can collect the knowledge of the best experts and the latest reports from labs around the world for use by physicians at any hospital, clinic, or independent practice.

**DXplain** is another decision support system that is commercially available to clinicians. The name is based on the medical shorthand for diagnosis: Dx. Like GIDEON and other similar systems, DXplain takes in information from a patient's medical history, physical findings, and results from tests and scans. Then it offers a list of common and rare conditions to consider.

According to its designers, DXplain contains "over 4,800 clinical manifestations associated with over 2,200 different diseases." This system includes all sorts of conditions, not just infectious diseases. Physicians can work forward or backward, either entering clinical findings to see what diseases might be present, or putting in a suspected disease in order to see what signs and symptoms may be present.

Researchers at the Mayo Clinic in Rochester, Minnesota, surveyed a group of medical students who had access to DXplain as they did their rounds. Almost three out of four of the medical students said the computer system frequently or always suggested diagnoses they had not considered. And the rest of the students said DXplain offered a novel diagnosis at least some of the time. Most of the medical students said they would like to have the decision support system regularly available.

**UpToDate** is a popular computer-based resource for physicians that is intended to help them get answers quickly during the hectic demands of clinical practice. It is overseen by a collection of medical societies. Several independent surveys highlighted on the UpToDate web site (www.uptodate.com) report that the system is frequently used by many physicians and is often the most popular electronic reference source. Physicians told surveyors that they could usually get answers in less than fifteen minutes and that frequently they could avoid having to consult with a specialist. Most of the physicians in several of the surveys said that they had changed their diagnosis or treatment of their patients based on the information they learned by using the UpToDate computer system.

---

Professor Coiera created an online directory of artificial intelligence systems that are being studied or used in clinical applications. The work of maintaining the directory at www.openclinical.org has been continued by others. The section on artificial intelligence systems in clinical practice now includes dozens of different applications, not only helping physicians and others make diagnoses but also offering support in acute care, using and interpreting laboratory tests and medical imaging, managing clinical practice, and educating both patients and students in health care professions.

Decision support software is spreading beyond physicians. There is a growing number of web-based systems oriented toward patients. For instance, one such web site allows patients to enter very specific details about their cancer, whether it is melanoma or breast cancer, prostate cancer, or several other types. The system takes the lab and clinical reports and the patient's own assessment of his or her health and then offers suggestions about what type of treatment might be considered as well as research trials that might be available. Of course, the system does not make medical recommendations. It is intended to be an educational tool that helps people sort through vast amounts of cancer treatment information to find the parts that are most relevant to their specific type of cancer.

There is a variety of tools for people concerned about their risk of developing heart disease. They use recommendations from expert groups and summaries of research in an attempt to provide individualized predictions based on factors such as age, cholesterol, blood pressure, and smoking. For instance, one such heart disease risk calculator factors in the potential benefits—and risks—of certain preventive actions, such as taking aspirin or medications that can reduce cholesterol or blood pressure. Of course, everyone who visits the site is advised to avoid smoking, eat better, and incorporate more physical activity in their daily routines.

As such web-based systems proliferate, they do raise questions about credibility and expertise. Someone going to a physician knows the doctor is licensed and perhaps has a certificate from a professional board showing that he or she has demonstrated some expertise in a particular specialty. But anyone can create a web site, and there is not necessarily any connection between how sophisticated the site appears to be and the underlying value of the information or advice it provides. Patients are in many ways left to fend for themselves . . . and check to see who is supplying the information for a web site, whether it is a public agency or university, or perhaps a private company with products to sell, or even an individual.

---

### Whither the Stethoscope?

Computers are infiltrating even that most iconic badge of the physician: the stethoscope.

The stethoscope "embodies the essence of doctoring: using science and technology in concert with the human skill of listening to determine what ails a patient," according to a perspective piece in the *New England Journal of Medicine* written by Howard Markel, M.D., Ph.D. He is the director of the Center for the History of Medicine at the University of Michigan Medical School in Ann Arbor.

However, the stethoscope may be turning into more of a symbol than a regular tool, at least in its classic form. There are now electronic stethoscopes that take over some of the listening and interpreting of sounds in patients' bodies.

The online brochure for one such device boasts that "When combined with the 3M Sound Analysis Software you have an exquisite, state-of-the-art auscultation system, which allows you to see what you are hearing via visual display of a phonocardiogram. This hardware and software combination will enhance teaching opportunities, serve as a diagnostic aid and help you make more effective use of telemedicine."

This particular model runs a bit more than $400, compared to $100 or so for a classic stethoscope. The physician can still listen through this hybrid model, but other digital stethoscopes do all the listening electronically, using microphones or ultrasound to gather data for analysis.

In one research study, an electronic stethoscope was used to feed data to a computer program that used a neural network type of artificial intelligence. In this test, the electronic system was asked to distinguish between patients who had serious heart disease and others who had heart murmurs that were considered harmless. The computer got a perfect score.

The researchers wrote that such a system could be used for high-volume screening of children to pick out early signs of heart disease.

While many physicians turn wistful when recalling their first stethoscope and cling to it as a link to medical tradition, in a way the modern technological assault facing stethoscopes is fitting. When the stethoscope was first introduced, it faced many skeptics, including physicians who rejected the device as a radical departure from the time-honored practice of putting one's ear to the chest of the patient.

A recent commentary posted on a web site of the British National Health Service quoted a negative review of stethoscopes that appeared in the London *Times* in 1834. "That it will ever come into general use, notwithstanding its value, is extremely doubtful; because its beneficial application requires much time and gives a good bit of trouble both to the patient and the practitioner; because its hue and character are foreign and opposed to all our habits and associations," the newspaper reported.

And medical historian Dr. Markel notes that in hindsight, the seeds of the stethoscope's possible demise could be seen at its birth. "After all, its creation initiated an irreversible trend in medicine by physically separating diagnosing physicians from their patients, albeit only by the length of a hollow tube," Dr. Markel wrote.

---

Medical technology marches forward. But while the latest laboratory test and imaging studies, along with older techniques of physical examination and history taking, provide essential pieces of information, they do not, by themselves, diagnose patients. Even with a computer assist, it is up to physicians to pull together all the known facts, judge the credibility and relevance of the findings, and then select the best explanation from the range of possible diagnoses. That's where Dr. House's whiteboard comes into play.

# FIVE

# The Whiteboard

Much of the medical action on *House, M.D.* occurs in exam rooms, in the lab, at the bedside, and in treatment rooms . . . but the heart of Dr. House's work is found in the "diagnosis room." This generous conference area is home to his whiteboard. On this board, Dr. House and his team list the patient's symptoms and signs . . . often alongside possible diagnoses. The whiteboard is the essence of the show. The concise notations written on the board distill and track each case from presentation to resolution.

Although few physicians have their own private conference rooms, every physician relies on a process like that embodied by the whiteboard. "Differential diagnosis" is the logical exercise during which clinical signs and symptoms are compared to possible diagnoses. In most cases, the diagnosis is fairly straightforward.

There is almost always more than one possible explanation for a patient's chief complaint, even if one diagnosis is far more likely than others. For instance, a patient with cough, headache, and muscle pain probably has the flu . . . but the "differentials" include a number of other infections with bacteria, fungi, or other viruses. As we discussed earlier, young physicians are trained to look for the most likely suspects suggested by the symptoms and signs; that is, that horses, not zebras, are probably the source of the hoofbeats they hear. Emergency room physicians are trained to quickly investigate the most lethal diagnoses. For instance, chest pain could be caused by a tear in the aorta, which can kill in minutes. Heart attack is more likely, but not as deadly or swift. Muscle strain and heartburn are the most common, but least dangerous, diagnoses.

Such cases are dismissed by Dr. House as banal and unworthy of his attention. Each episode of *House, M.D.* builds around a case full of twists and turns that shatter expectations, whether it's a tapeworm in a young woman's brain, a mutant measles viral time bomb, or a genetic disorder masquerading as mental illness. The cases are bizarre, indeed. But while they may seem almost too fantastic, weird things do happen.

And though a relatively manageable list of infectious and chronic diseases, metabolic disorders, and genetic abnormalities explain the overwhelming majority of cases, F. Parkes Weber, M.D., is credited with pointing out that, "For one common disease or syndrome there are several rare ones." In other words, each rare condition is by itself rare, but when all the rare conditions are added together, it is not really that unusual to come across something strange. As one veteran emergency physician put it, he is surprised every shift and completely stumped by a case monthly.

Whether a particular case is a "stumper" or mundane, the process of generating differentials and then ruling them out is essentially the same. One article on the art of diagnosis described six basic steps: grouping the clinical findings into patterns, selecting a key finding, listing the possible causes, pruning that list, selecting a diagnosis, and then validating that diagnosis. An important skill is the ability to cast a net wide enough to catch the actual diagnosis, without endlessly chasing unlikely causes. What's more, these critical choices must be made in the face of incomplete evidence.

> Because the properties of the individual items of history and physical examination often are not available, you must rely on clinical experience and intuition to predict the extent to which many pieces of information modify your differential diagnosis. For some clinical problems, including the diagnosis of pulmonary embolism, clinicians' intuition has proved remarkably accurate.
>
> —*Users' Guides to the Medical Literature*, American Medical Association

In "Daddy's Boy" (2-05), the patient was a young man who had just finished college. At a party he suddenly suffered an attack of shocklike sensations. In addition, he had headaches, nausea, and drowsiness. The initial whiteboard list had just those symptoms listed.

A formal case presentation of the type used in medical education is typically far more detailed. The whiteboard (indeed the findings and causes are often listed on a whiteboard in a medical school or hospital conference room) would usually list all the key characteristics of the patient and the findings from examinations and tests, albeit in medical shorthand. Also there would be a column listing causes that the physicians making the presentation consider to be among the differential diagnoses.

On the show, Wilson, Dr. House, and the rest of the team quickly ran through a number of possible causes. In reality, the list might be quite long.

For example, multiple sclerosis was briefly mentioned by Cameron. The differential diagnoses for multiple sclerosis include about two dozen other diseases and syndromes, ranging from infections attacking the nervous system to growths in the brain, from opportunistic infections due to HIV/AIDS to inherited metabolic disorders, from blood vessel disorders to Lyme disease.

Lupus also is on lists of differential diagnoses for multiple sclerosis. There are specific tests that can be done to either rule in or rule out the disease. One of the most common is called an ANA, which is short for an antinuclear antibody test. Blood is drawn in order to check for the presence of antibodies that attack the patient's own cells. If the antibodies attack nerve cells, then neurological disorders may be the result.

The ANA test results would be added to the list of findings. But as with most tests, this single piece of information is unlikely to settle things. Almost all patients with lupus have a positive ANA test result. However, about one in twenty does not, so a negative test does not necessarily mean the patient is free of lupus. On the other hand, a positive result does not always indicate lupus. In fact, a positive ANA result may suggest one of several kinds of autoimmune disorders, including Sjögren's syndrome, which is a systemic inflammatory disease, or scleroderma or other related rheumatic diseases.

In addition to test results that add more information to the list on the whiteboard, time often provides more clues. In this particular case on *House, M.D.*, the patient developed sphincter paralysis. That event prompted Foreman to suggest Miller Fisher syndrome, which is a variety of Guillain-Barré syndrome. These syndromes tend to occur after an infection. Patients suffer symptoms related to an autoimmune attack that damages nerve cells. They have abnormal or weak muscle action and certain forms of paralysis, which may progress to a dangerous level.

There was a spike in the number of Guillain-Barré syndrome cases in the United States in 1976 after people were vaccinated against swine flu. There are some anecdotal reports of cases after other vaccinations, but scientific studies have not reported evidence of a link between Guillain-Barré syndrome and any immunizations other than the 1976 swine flu vaccine.

Since the causes of Guillain-Barré syndrome and the Miller Fisher syndrome are poorly understood, these syndromes are hard to either prove or disprove. As a result, they may linger on the whiteboard's list of potential causes, while other possible diagnoses are investigated.

Guillain-Barré syndrome and Miller Fisher syndrome have their own lists of differential diagnoses, which overlap with multiple sclerosis and other causes of neurological disorders. Clinicians may look for signs of paraneoplastic syndromes, which would point to an underlying cancer.

David N. Gilbert, M.D., director of Medical Education at Providence Portland Medical Center in Portland, Oregon, and coeditor of *The Sanford Guide to Antimicrobial Therapy*, describes differential diagnosis as an "ever-branching tree." One possible diagnosis may suggest several more and so on and so on. Dr. Gilbert says that as physicians gain experience they develop skill at recognizing patterns that help them to make sense of the fragmentary clues the patient brings them. Is the complaint acute or chronic? Is it progressing quickly or slowly? Is it an inflammatory process or not?

The branches of differential diagnoses could be followed to infinity, if clinicians did not impose some limits on the process. Diseases that are the most common naturally get attention. The consequences of conditions and the available treatments also get factored in. These judgments become second nature to experienced physicians.

"Whenever you construct a differential diagnosis, the good doctors put at the end of the list: 'or it could be something else I haven't thought of just yet,'" says Dr. John Sotos, the author of *Zebra Cards*, a book that helps physicians become familiar with the signs and symptoms of unfamiliar conditions.

"As you go through the evaluation, if things just don't fit right, you've got to start expanding your list. What you don't want to do is fall in love with an initial hypothesis and attempt to make all of the patients' manifestations fit into that hypothesis. That's intellectually dishonest and it does a disservice to the patient. You'll make errors. You've got to be dispassionate, look at the evidence, and see what fits. And when it starts to not fit, then you've got to cast your net a little wider," he says.

One critical skill is deciding when a finding that doesn't seem to fit the pattern is significant and when it is just a distraction. Dr. Sotos says there isn't a bright line or a single moment where such a decision is made. The differential diagnosis list evolves as new information becomes available.

Dr. Sotos underlines the difference between how experienced clinicians work and the type of formal differential diagnosis session you might see in a conference room at an academic medical center.

"I would describe it as a teaching exercise. It is very artificial. It is for inexperienced people. That exercise morphs over time into more of a pattern-matching process," he says. Nevertheless, even veteran doctors may fall back on a more formal process if they have to venture beyond the routine scope of their practice or specialty. "Even somebody very experienced at, say, neurology, when all of a sudden presented with a case involving obstetrics, is going to retreat to that slow and deliberate process."

Dr. Sotos says that even though the whiteboard is featured prominently in each episode of *House, M.D.*, Dr. House often jumps ahead, making quick decisions about what test or treatment should be tried next, decisions that often are not explained until later.

---

## The Art of Medicine

When a patient poses challenging clinical problems, an effective physician must be able to identify the crucial elements in a complex history and physical examination and extract the key laboratory results from the crowded computer printouts of data in order to determine whether to "treat" or to "watch." Deciding whether a clinical clue is worth pursuing or should be dismissed as a "red herring" and weighing whether a proposed treatment entails a greater risk than the disease itself are essential judgments that the skilled clinician must make many times each day. This combination of medical knowledge, intuition, experience, and judgment defines the art of medicine, which is as necessary to the practice of medicine as is a sound scientific base.

*—Harrison's Principles of Internal Medicine,* 16th edition

---

As we noted earlier when discussing evaluations in an emergency room, a tear in the aorta gets serious consideration when a patient complains of chest pain, even though it is relatively rare, because it can kill quickly. An uncommon condition may also get a closer look if there is an effective treatment available, even if the consequences of the disease are not immediately dire. On the other hand, if there is no effective treatment for a condition, then it may be put lower on the list of possible causes to check out, since a delay would not necessarily change the ultimate outcome for the patient.

For example, when a person comes to a doctor complaining of involuntary muscle movements and rigidity, one possible cause is Huntington's Disease. This inherited disorder is rare, affecting only about one person in 20,000 in most western nations. Huntington's is eventually deadly, but the progression can take longer than a decade. There is no known cure.

But the initial complaint of movement problems that might suggest possible Huntington's disease could also be caused by Parkinson's disease, which can be managed by treatment for an extended period.

Another possibility is Wilson's disease, which is a disorder related to how the body processes copper. Wilson's disease can be managed through a careful diet and medication. So a physician may well chase down the diagnostic branch leading toward Wilson's disease first, since starting the patient on a low-copper diet may prevent progression of the condition.

---

## The Eyes Have It

A thirty-eight-year-old mother acts strangely. She drinks and has signs of liver damage. So the diagnosis of schizophrenia and alcoholism she has early in the episode "The Socratic Method" (1-06) seems reasonable. Yet House doubts the easy answer, of course, and eventually a notation about a missed eye doctor appointment leads him to a diagnosis of Wilson's disease, a genetic disorder that leads to a damaging overload of copper in the body.

House suspected that the patient's psychiatric symptoms might not be schizophrenia, and with good reason. There is a very long list of conditions that may be confused with schizophrenia. So when he reviewed notes taken by the patient's son and saw that she had skipped an eye doctor appointment, it would be only natural to wonder what the results of an eye exam might have revealed.

Greenish-gold rings in the cornea of the eye are a classic sign of Wilson's disease, though they are not always obvious. A routine exam of the patient's eyes using a slit lamp will often highlight these rings of copper and sulfur granules. These deposits are called Kayser-Fleischer rings.

In actual practice, any patient suspected of having schizophrenia probably would be checked for Wilson's, because specific and effective treatment is available. Certainly it seems that prominent Kayser-Fleischer rings should not have been missed.

Liver scarring is also a sign of Wilson's. The genetic disorder impairs the body's ability to regulate its levels of copper. The resulting excess of copper damages the liver first and as copper levels rise, some escapes into the blood circulation and is deposited in other organs. Any patient with unexplained liver disease should be checked for Wilson's. Liver failure is the most lethal feature of the disorder.

One question raised by the episode is why the patient would have sought an eye exam. Chase suggests cataracts. Cataracts, a clouding of the lens of the eye, do indeed occur in people with Wilson's disease. However, the type usually linked to Wilson's, called sunflower cataracts, usually don't limit vision, making it less likely that they would be the reason to seek an eye exam.

The first-line treatment for Wilson's disease involves chelating agents that bind to excess copper, so that the body can excrete it more easily, along with dietary changes to limit copper intake.

## Thresholds

Few things in life or medicine are absolutely certain, so clinicians also organize their diagnostic investigations around test and treatment thresholds. When something is below the test threshold, it means that particular cause is so unlikely that it is not worth testing for, even if it is not completely impossible. At the other end of the spectrum, if a possible cause exceeds the treatment threshold, it means the probability is high enough to go ahead with treatment, even if the physician cannot offer a 100 percent guarantee.

There are formulas for calculating the test and treatment thresholds, though physicians may approach them more informally. The calculations, precise or intuitive, include both the benefits and the potential harms of tests and treatments.

For instance, in very rare cases, the first symptom of a brain tumor is a headache. But physicians do not order an MRI exam of every patient who comes in with a throbbing temple. The MRI may not be hazardous in most cases, but the test is expensive and it is unlikely to produce any useful information for the headache sufferer. Even if cost were not an issue, health care professionals are responsible for the wise use of medical resources. Testing everyone might mean long waits and a potentially hazardous delay for patients for whom the test results might be crucial.

Or consider all the blood tests available. How many times do you really want a needle stuck in your veins to draw more serum for testing? Beyond the minor pain of a blood draw, there is always the risk of a false positive result; that is, some tests will come back positive even when the patient does not actually have the thing being tested for. For example, PSA blood tests that are intended to detect signs of prostate cancer may show elevated levels of the prostate-specific antigen for a variety of reasons. The next step after a confirming the high PSA blood test result is often a needle biopsy procedure to retrieve tissue samples from the prostate. While the needle biopsy test may confirm the presence of cancer, in most cases, no tumor is found.

So the question facing men and their physician is: When is it worthwhile to undergo the discomfort and anxiety of a needle biopsy procedure? That question is not always easy to answer . . . and the answer may be different for different men, depending on their personal views.

A similar balancing of risks and benefits must be done with treatments. How certain do you have to be before starting therapy? It depends.

If the disease is dangerous and the treatment reasonably safe, then the treatment threshold may be very low. For example, patients who come to an emergency room with chest pain may be given aspirin long before doctors are certain that a heart attack is under way, because rapid treatment with aspirin can help restore blood flow to the heart muscle, thus limiting the damage of the heart attack. Aspirin can cause bleeding in the stomach or intestines, but the danger is relatively low, especially for a patient being monitored in an emergency department.

But going back to the prostate cancer example, that treatment threshold is higher. The most common treatment for prostate cancer is surgery to remove the prostate gland. The surgery is not only painful, but many patients also suffer long-term or even permanent incontinence and impotence. No one would rush into surgery on the basis of just a PSA blood test. Even after a needle biopsy procedure is done—and cancer is confirmed—there may be questions about whether the treatment threshold has been crossed. If the cancer has already spread beyond the prostate, surgery probably won't help the patient because it won't remove all the cancer. Also, prostate tumors tend to grow very slowly; tumors can take years or even decades to cause health problems. An elderly man with other health problems may decide to skip the surgery, even if he has cancer, figuring that surgery to remove a small tumor may not provide benefits that outweigh the trauma of the operation and its aftermath.

In general, Dr. House's test threshold is nearly zero. If there is any chance at all of finding something, he tends to order another blood draw, a lumbar puncture, MRI, CT scan, and so on. He also demonstrates a low treatment threshold, often starting therapy well before he is confident of his diagnosis. The risks of tests and procedures rarely dissuade him.

Perhaps the most extreme example is from the episode "Autopsy" (2-02). Dr. House said the only way to prove the existence of a suspected clot inside the brain of young patient would be to chill her body until it essentially shuts down and then drain the blood from her brain and return it while tracking the flow via MRI. The drastic step of hypothermic arrest is sometimes used to reduce the hazards of surgery on the brain or its major arteries. Brain tissue can survive longer without normal blood flow when it is cold. That phenomenon explains the survival of some people who have been revived after being submerged in icy waters. Taking such extreme steps to minimize the risk of a treatment procedure is one thing. Subjecting a patient to a very dangerous procedure in order to confirm a diagnosis is something else.

Sometimes it is hardest to pare the differential diagnosis list when the symptoms are the most commonplace. Fatigue or a general feeling of tiredness is one of the most common complaints and also one of the most difficult to pin down. The differential diagnosis list may include hypothyroidism, diabetes, anemia, mononucleosis, depression, and more.

"I'll work up the patient and I may think the most probable diagnosis here, based on everything I know, is anemia. So that's my working diagnosis. But I'm going to keep all of these other diagnoses in the back of my head; I'm not going to just throw them out. I'm going to keep thinking about all of them," says family practice physician Rick Kellerman, M.D.

But if working through the list doesn't lead to a prime suspect, Dr. Kellerman says he may seek a second opinion, both to tap another physician's expertise about the possible underlying cause of the complaint, and also to check to see how urgent the problem seems to be. Is there time to do more testing? Or is one of the suspects lingering on the differential diagnosis list dangerous enough to justify treatment, even before absolute proof of the real cause is available?

Barreling ahead with treatment, before all the facts are in, is a frequent occurrence on *House, M.D.* In one episode, Dr. House ordered treatment for Guillain-Barré syndrome, even though the antibody tests for the disease were negative. He suspected the test might have just missed something. Since he believed that the treatment of plasmapheresis, which is a type of blood filtering, and intravenous immunoglobulin G presented little risk of side effects, it made sense to proceed. If the treatment worked, it would support the Guillain-Barré syndrome diagnosis . . . and if it didn't help, they could look harder at other possibilities.

---

## Too Much of a Good Thing

In the early stages of investigating a case, Dr. House frequently prescribes an array of antibiotics. His thinking is that if the disease is a bacterial infection, the antibiotics will help, and even if the problem is something else, well, most antibiotics have few side effects, so what's the harm?

Actually, overreliance on antibiotics has created a serious threat to our ability to fight infectious diseases. The problem is that the microbes are evolving and becoming resistant to antibiotics and other antimicrobial agents. According to the Centers for Disease Control and Prevention (CDC), nearly 2 million patients in the United States catch a bug while they are in the hospital and about 90,000 die as a result of their infection.

Hospitals are havens for microbes. After all, hospitals are full of sick people, including many who are vulnerable to infections because they have weakened immune systems. To make matters worse, many of the microbes in hospitals are like hardened criminals in maximum-security prisons: They know all the tricks and they can be ruthless in using them. More than 70 percent of the bacteria that cause infections in hospitals are resistant to at least one of the drugs most commonly used to treat them, the CDC reports.

Some microbes are becoming resistant to several drugs. A report in the journal *Clinical Infectious Diseases* said that in 1992, just over a third of *Staphylococcus aureus* infections in hospital intensive care units were resistant to several important drugs. By 2003, almost two-thirds of the *Staphylococcus aureus* samples collected in ICUs were resistant to multiple drugs. There is growing concern about superbugs that might not be treatable with any drugs that are currently available. Adding to that concern is the small number of new drugs being tested.

Some experts warn that the future may look like the days before antibiotics, when physicians had no effective weapons against common microbes. Patients either got better on their own . . . or they didn't. There are worldwide campaigns under way to forestall that frightening prospect. A key feature of these campaigns is advice to physicians and their patients to resist the urge to casually prescribe antibiotics when an infection is suspected. The hope is that by using antimicrobial drugs carefully, researchers will have more time to develop new tools to keep us a step ahead of the constantly evolving microbes.

---

Starting treatment in order to help pare down the differential diagnosis list, while also possibly helping the patient, is a variation of the concept of a treatment threshold. That is, physicians frequently cannot wait to know the cause of a patient's complaint with 100 percent certainty. If there is at least a reasonable basis for suspecting a certain cause, and if the side effects and other risks of treatment appear to be acceptable, then the fact that beginning a treatment may either help prove or disprove the preliminary diagnosis is one more item that can tip the scale in favor of going ahead with treatment.

Of course, then the physician needs to monitor the effects of therapy in order to determine if the treatment is the right course. In the episode "DNR" (1-09), the patient was receiving several treatments at the same time. When he started getting better, there was no way to tell which treatment was responsible. In this case, Dr. House recommended stopping everything, and then adding back one treatment at a time. That way, they could identify which treatment was helping and which were doing nothing.

## Doing Nothing

Then there are the cases where doing nothing is the wisest course, at least for a while.

"Tincture of time" is the phrase many doctors use to refer to those cases in which it turns out that inaction, at least for a little while, is the best action.

"Say I can't figure out what it is. The tests look okay. It's not a serious problem, doesn't look like something the patient could die from," Dr. Kellerman says. "One of the things we do then, one of our best and most cost-effective tests, is to give it a little bit of time. Not years, of course, but you've done a good workup and you want to wait a week or two and see what happens. Some things, due to viruses, stress, who knows what, go away and the patient feels better. We may never know exactly what it was."

There is no hard and fast rule about how long to wait for an illness to either resolve itself or show its true colors, but physicians and patients are often rewarded by patience.

In the first episode of *House, M.D.*, even Dr. House, despite his typically impatient temperament, recommended waiting, although the patient's condition was quite serious. In this case, the causes near the top of the differential diagnosis list each had very different rates of progression. So Dr. House decided that if he just watched, the true cause would reveal itself. The speed of the patient's decline then did rule out cancer. Eventually, the team found evidence that a tapeworm had infected the patient's brain and other organs.

## Neurocysticercosis

Tapeworm cysts in the brains of patients are rare in the United States, but they seem to be occurring more frequently, even among people who have never traveled to foreign countries where the parasitic infections are more common. Cysticercosis is caused by the larval stage of a tapeworm found in pigs, *Taenia solium*. About a thousand cases are reported in the United States each year. About one case in ten may be neurocysticercosis, which means that cysts have developed in the brain or spinal column.

As in the first episode of *House, M.D.*, the first symptom of neurocysticercosis is often a seizure. And there may be nothing obvious to suggest a tapeworm. In fact, four cases were reported among orthodox Jews in New York, who never ate or handled pork. Investigators determined the parasites were probably transmitted by domestic workers who helped make meals.

Sometimes the source of the parasites is never found. When a healthy six-year-old girl living in a suburb of Chicago had a seizure, her doctors began treatment for what they thought were brain abscesses. During surgery on her brain, doctors discovered that what looked like an abscess was actually a cyst containing a partially degenerated tapeworm larva. The only trip outside the United States that the girl had ever taken was to Ireland, where tapeworms are uncommon. Nothing that would indicate parasites was seen in stool samples from the girl or other members of the family.

Tapeworm infections are usually diagnosed by using immune system tests that find signs of an antibody reaction to parasites. CT scans, MRIs, and eye exams may also help doctors find evidence of the cysts. A simple bedpan check will often reveal evidence of tapeworms, but not always, as the case of the girl in Chicago shows.

In the pilot episode, House's team did not scan the patient's brain, although such scans can show tapeworm cysts in the brain. However, when brain scans are not available, physicians do sometimes X-ray other parts of the body to look for evidence of parasites, just as Chase suggested.

Albendazole is one of the drugs typically used to treat serious cases of neurocysticercosis. The drug can reduce the frequency and severity of seizures, but it may not eliminate them entirely.

---

Dr. Gilbert notes that waiting and watching were once more common, whereas the typical response to uncertainty today is to order more tests and scans.

"Doctors used to wait for more signs and symptoms to become evident," Dr. Gilbert says. "Time can be your friend and often the smartest thing to do is to wait."

He recalls a young woman he saw in the 1970s. She wasn't feeling well and a throat culture came back positive for strep. He prescribed antibiotics, but instead of feeling better, she got worse. Her throat was raw. Tests of her kidney function seemed a bit odd. Dr. Gilbert didn't know what the cause of her symptoms was, but it wasn't strep. He stopped the antibiotic treatment, since it clearly was not helping. He referred her on to other physicians.

Years later he and his former patient again crossed paths. She looked different. The bridge of her nose had flattened. A saddle nose can be a sign of a disease called Wegener's granulomatosis, which is an unusual blood vessel problem in which inflamed vessels starve certain tissues of blood flow.

Wegener's granulomatosis had never made it onto Dr. Gilbert's original list of differential diagnoses. There are no blood tests that would specifically identify Wegener's granulomatosis. Eventually, the woman had a biopsy of the affected area, which is the primary method for diagnosing the disease. Medical therapy can usually help, although many patients have a recurrence.

"Based on what I saw when she first came to me it would have seemed impossible," he says. "But time brought out other symptoms."

In many places in the world, where high-tech imaging machines are not just down the hall, waiting and watching to see which symptoms appear in which order and at what rate is still a key diagnostic tactic.

Of course, some cases are never solved. One study of more than a thousand patients who came to an ear, nose, and throat clinic complaining of dizziness found that about one out of four remained undiagnosed.

Fever is another symptom that can frustrate physicians and patients alike. Indeed, so many doctors have been stumped by cases involving persistent fevers that the situation earned its own name, "FUO," which is short for fever of unknown origin. The classic definition is fever persisting for more than three weeks, documented temperature above 101°F on several occasions, and an uncertain diagnosis after extensive evaluation in the hospital for one week. The actual causes of those cases that are eventually resolved range from infections to tumors to vascular disease, with other miscellaneous causes thrown into the mix.

The types of cases involving fever that torment physicians seem to have changed in recent years. When underlying causes are eventually discovered, cancer is less likely to be the explanation than it was in previous decades. Researchers say they suspect several factors are involved in this shift, but they suspect advances in diagnostic technology, such as ultrasound and CT scans mean tumors are more likely to be detected before a case gets tagged with the FUO label.

But even in the face of tremendous technological progress, as many as one out of three cases of fever of unknown origin is never completely figured out. These patients get better on their own and the illnesses simply remain mysteries. Unfortunately, some cases that are puzzles at first later reveal deadly causes. In one series of patients, cancer in the blood was responsible for about one in ten cases of what had been fever of unknown origin. However, these blood diseases, particularly non-Hodgkin's lymphoma, accounted for more than half the deaths recorded by the researchers.

Disease often tells its secrets in a casual parenthesis.

—Wilfred Batten Lewis Trotter (1872–1939)

Dr. House should probably give recognition to pioneering British cancer surgeon and neurosurgeon Wilfred Trotter. The cases he and his team tackle don't shout out their solutions. They drop whispered hints that are heard only through careful listening. And yet when the subtle clues are recognized, they often bring a sharp change in the direction of the diagnostic inquiry.

"It's that off-hand remark that the patient makes that turns on the lightbulb. If the patient presents with syndrome 'A' and their presentation is wholly compatible with syndrome 'A,' so you are thinking syndrome 'A,' and then they just make a remark like, 'Oh, yeah, my toes turn blue when that happens.' It's something they pay no attention to, they really don't understand the significance of it, but all of a sudden it causes you immediately to pull up stakes and shift to syndrome 'B,'" says Dr. John Sotos, who quoted Dr. Trotter in his book on uncommon diseases and presentations, *Zebra Cards*.

In the first episode of *House, M.D.*, the plot turned on a casual remark by Foreman about eating a ham sandwich at the patient's apartment. Suddenly a food-borne parasite jumped on to the differential diagnosis list.

In the "Daddy's Boy" episode discussed earlier in this chapter, the patient's most dramatic early sign was shock-like sensations. None of the early suspects panned out. But then Dr. House suddenly dropped everything and sprang into action when a friend of the patient made a seemingly casual remark about the boy's summer job in his father's junkyard. The "casual parenthesis" contained a key clue: that the patient's ailment might be linked to something found in scrap-metal yards. A search of the boy's belongings then turned up a seemingly unremarkable metal bauble. The piece of scrap was hardly innocuous. It was radioactive.

Although radiation poisoning did not appear on the whiteboard until late in this episode, perhaps it should have. Early on, Cameron mentioned that the shocks could be Lhermitte's sign, which is sometimes an early symptom of multiple sclerosis. However, multiple sclerosis is not the only cause. Lhermitte's sign can also be caused by radiation exposure. In fact, the shock sensation is a common consequence of radiation therapy.

## Heuristics

Although medicine is increasingly scientific, physicians are human . . . and as they grapple with the evidence available in a difficult case, human nature can lead them down the wrong path. Analysis of the way people make sense of the world around reveals that we often take logical shortcuts in order to reach a decision.

These shortcuts are part of the reason experienced physicians can rapidly arrive at a diagnosis without plodding through each step of a complete examination and formal differential diagnosis process the way they did as young interns or residents.

Every profession has its "rules of thumb," strategies based on experience of what usually works and what doesn't. A technical term for a rule of thumb is a heuristic. One example of a popular heuristic is Occam's razor, the belief that when several solutions are possible, the simplest one is preferred. Most of the time heuristics improve our efficiency. They allow us to make decisions even when the evidence is incomplete or confusing. It's natural that people rely on these strategies when we are in a hurry . . . and doctors trying to decide on a diagnosis are almost always in a hurry.

Despite their enormous practical utility, heuristics can also take us quickly in the wrong direction.

Three decades ago, Amos Tversky and Daniel Kahneman wrote an oft-quoted paper that appeared in the journal *Science*, titled "Judgment under Uncertainty: Heuristics and Biases." The authors offered a model of how people make decisions even though we often don't have all the facts. They proposed almost a dozen types of biases or "cognitive illusions" that can affect judgment.

The model has its critics, who question how accurately it captures human decision-making in the real world. Nevertheless, the famous paper and subsequent articles and books had a profound influence on popular concepts of human thinking processes, particularly medical diagnosis. Certainly, physicians have to be aware of, and try to counterbalance, the natural human tendency to jump to conclusions. Indeed, that training in critical thinking underlies much medical education.

## THE AVAILABILITY HEURISTIC

If you saw or heard about something recently, you are more likely to think of it when faced with similar circumstances.

"These heuristics can be inimical to the process of diagnosis. So some institutions will train their medical students and residents to recognize when they are being lured down a false path by one of these heuristics, including the Availability heuristic. If I saw a case of alkaptonuria last week, I am much more likely to diagnose it this week because of the Availability heuristic: Things that happened recently stick in the mind," Dr. Sotos says.

Alkaptonuria is a rare inherited metabolic disorder that can be one cause of discolored urine, but it occurs in less than one person in 25,000.

Of course, *House, M.D.* is rooted in the premise that just because something is extremely unlikely does not mean it is not the cause of a particular case. Indeed, many seasoned physicians can recall cases in which a medical student chooses a rare disease as the explanation for a patient's symptoms. And sometimes, says Dr. Sotos, the young doctor turns out to be right.

"He finishes his presentation and says, 'I think this is a clear case of reticulum cell sarcoma,' which is an incredibly rare disease and everybody laughs at him. It turns out a week later that the patient does have reticulum cell sarcoma. They asked the student, 'How did you know that?!' He says, 'Well, what else causes splenomegaly?' Of course, there are a million things that can cause an enlarged spleen, but that was the only one he knew," Dr. Sotos says.

The "availability" or the amount of popular attention paid to something can also affect common perceptions about various health threats. Here's a pop quiz: Name the cancer that kills the most women in the United States each year. If you answered breast cancer, you have a lot of company. But the right answer is lung cancer. According to the American Cancer Society 2006 estimates, lung cancer kills over 72,000 women a year compared to about 41,000 deaths due to breast cancer. But in part because breast cancer gets much more public and media attention than lung cancer, many people assume it is the bigger killer.

## THE REPRESENTATIVENESS HEURISTIC

Additional information helps physicians make the right diagnosis, doesn't it? Well, not always. Sometimes the extra information can be a distraction and obscure important facts.

The Representativeness heuristic is what leads us to assume that someone who belongs to a certain group shares characteristics with others of that group. In a medical context, this heuristic can lead a doctor to either overestimate or underestimate the likelihood of a particular diagnosis.

At the beginning of "Daddy's Boy," when Dr. House heard that the patient was a college student who had just graduated, he quickly assumed that the complaint had something to do with heavy partying. He extrapolated his concept of the group, graduating college students, to the individual, who was actually sick from an entirely unrelated cause.

Occupation is a key fact that any physician wants to know about her patient. But she has to be careful not to allow the Representativeness heuristic to inflate the importance of that one fact and blind her to other clues.

Say an international aid worker who travels frequently to Africa and a local caterer come to the hospital complaining of vomiting, diarrhea, fatigue, and fever. It may be natural to assume that the causes are different; presuming that the aid worker is exposed to any number of exotic pathogens and the caterer spends most of the workday in the kitchen of his suburban home. So the aid worker gets checked for amoebas and other nasty critters, while the caterer is suspected of having salmonella bacteria from handling raw chicken.

But if the physicians working up those patients assumed that occupation was so important that they failed to ask each patient about their recent activities, including meals, they might not find out that both had partaken of the "Two-fer-a-Buck" raw oyster shooters at a bar in the hotel where the aid worker was staying, which also happened to be across the street from the office of the caterer's latest client. In this scenario, the oysters transmitted Norwalk virus from an infected kitchen worker. The complaints of the patients had nothing to do with their occupations.

## ANCHORING AND ADJUSTMENT

When trying to make estimates quickly or with incomplete information, where we start often influences where we end up.

For example, people tend to guess that a series of calculations that start with a large number will have a larger result than a similar series that begins with a small number. In one test, Tversky and Kahneman used the following equations:

$$1 \times 2 \times 3 \times 4 \times 5 \times 6 \times 7 \times 8 = ?$$
$$8 \times 7 \times 6 \times 5 \times 4 \times 3 \times 2 \times 1 = ?$$

People shown the equation starting with 1 gave much lower average estimates than did those shown the equation starting with 8, even though both yield the same result.

Another common way to see the effect of Anchoring and Adjustment on human judgment is to ask someone a question such as, "How common is the common cold? Do you think an estimate that 30 percent of people got a cold last winter is too high or too low?" Then ask someone else exactly the same question with this one change, "Do you think an estimate that 70 percent of people got a cold last winter is too high or too low?" In general, people's estimates of how many people really catch colds will be higher after given the second set of questions, because their minds latch onto the higher proposed estimate as a starting point.

A physician might have to resist the Anchoring and Adjustment pitfall depending on the order in which specific information or test results become available. For instance, if the result of a certain blood test leads the physician to believe the patient almost certainly has a certain disease, but then a second test casts doubt on that diagnosis, the physician may be more likely to stick with the original diagnosis than if the order of the tests was reversed, so that he received the result doubting the likelihood of the disease first.

## LOOKING FOR CONFIRMATION

A somewhat similar feature of human nature is the tendency to emphasize information that confirms our beliefs and to discount contradictory facts.

In the scenario of the caterer with stomach problems, if the doctor believed salmonella was the likely culprit, then the caterer's admission that, yes, he'd been handling raw chicken meat might carry a lot of weight; while at the same time the doctor might explain away news that the caterer's coworkers didn't get sick by assuming they had been more careful about washing their hands.

If the whiteboard has done its job of helping physicians organize all the information from examinations and tests—and then proposing and paring differential diagnoses suggested by the symptoms and signs—the result should be a diagnosis that exceeds the treatment threshold.

Of course, naming the disease isn't the end of the battle. The goal is preserving or restoring the health of the patient. Treatment aimed at cure or effective management of the condition is next.

# SIX

# Let's Make You Better

For Dr. House, the hunt is everything.

Standing at the whiteboard in "Daddy's Boy" (2-05), he says, "You're good, my friend, I'm sure we'll meet again." He's talking about the disease, not the patient. His focus is on making the right diagnosis; healing the patients that fill the hospital seems almost a fortunate by-product. For Dr. House, a happy ending means unmasking the disease. Of course, for patients the situation is exactly reversed. The cause is of less concern to them than the cure. Happy endings for patients mean successful treatments.

In "Control" (1-14), Dr. House did take some personal interest in the outcome of heart transplant surgery for his patient. The surgeon gave an upbeat report on the operation: "Textbook. She'll outlive us all."

Although not every patient on *House, M.D.* heads home with restored health, the team's batting average is enviable. Long life and full health is the most common prognosis, thanks to effective treatment made possible by the correct diagnosis. Actually, the odds of full recovery indeed may be relatively good for the type of patient featured on *House, M.D.*; that is, typically young and otherwise healthy, except for one little life-threatening oddity.

When the problem is some external exposure, such as a pesticide, or a treatable infection, or even a localized tumor, removing or eradicating the cause of the illnesses may well restore health. The same is true of trauma victims, such as people in car crashes, or those resuscitated quickly after nearly drowning. Once the crisis has passed, life can get back to almost normal after some rehabilitation.

Even the recipients of transplanted hearts often do well for years. The longest survivors have been living with their new hearts for more than twenty years. Among younger recipients (the patient in "Control" was said to be thirty-two years old), more than two out of three survive at least five years. One survey of heart transplant recipients about a decade after they got their new hearts found they were generally doing well. Of course, they have to keep taking immunosuppressive drugs to prevent rejection of the transplanted organs, and the long-term side effects of these drugs take a toll physically and emotionally.

---

## Ipecac & Broken Hearts

Syrup of ipecac was once a staple in home medicine cabinets. It was almost universally recommended as an emergency treatment to induce vomiting in someone who had swallowed poison.

But ipecac also has a history of abuse by people with eating disorders, such as bulimia nervosa. They use the drug to purge food from their stomachs after an eating binge. The eating disorder and purging behavior both are hard on the body. Ipecac adds its own hazards.

In the episode "Control" (1-14), a woman who was a hard-charging business executive was hiding her bulimia and ipecac abuse until heart damage almost killed her. There are a number of reports in the medical literature of severe damage or even deaths linked to ipecac abuse by people with eating disorders.

Ipecac is a plant native to South America. The word ipecac comes from the Tupi language of indigenous Indians in the region. With chronic use, ipecac damages muscle tissue. When the damage occurs in the heart muscle, it is called cardiomyopathy. The result can be heart failure.

According to the *Cecil Textbook of Medicine*, sudden death from cardiac failure is a risk of ipecac abuse. The textbook says death is uncommon, but firm numbers are hard to come by.

Since ipecac is sold over the counter, manufacturers do not have to report problems the way they would with a prescription drug, so there is no way to know exactly how many people have been harmed or killed by ipecac abuse. Still there are some case reports from poison centers and others. One presentation to the U.S. Food and Drug Administration, submitted as part of a review of ipecac's "over-the-counter" status in 2003, reported that of seventeen cases of ipecac toxicity that were investigated, six involved women with eating disorders who abused the drug. They ranged in age from nineteen to thirty-five. Five of the women exhibited signs of myopathy. One suffered cardiac arrest caused by emetine, one of the chemical components of ipecac.

Four of these women died from ipecac toxicity. One suffered permanent heart damage. Only one recovered.

People who abuse ipecac may have abnormal results on electrocardiograms or muscle enzyme tests. Ipecac can also be detected through tox screens of blood serum, urine, or tissue samples.

The patient on *House, M.D.* received a heart transplant because ipecac had caused irreparable damage to her heart. There are some reports in the medical literature that patients may recover from ipecac abuse, including one case of a patient whose heart function returned to normal within ten days after the abuse was stopped.

The author of the report to the FDA on ipecac damage and death recommended that further studies be done to see just how widespread the problem is. He also recommended changing the label on ipecac bottles to spell out the potentially serious risks and warn about abuse. He said the FDA should even consider requiring people to get a prescription for ipecac.

After discovering that ipecac abuse was causing his patient's heart damage, Dr. House told her how bad habitual use was, but he said the drug was great for getting a child to vomit after accidentally swallowing a bottle of aspirin.

The American Academy of Pediatrics, which for decades agreed with that outlook, changed its view in 2003. The academy adopted a new policy saying ipecac should no longer be kept in homes as an emergency treatment for poisonings.

"Although it seems to make sense to induce vomiting after the ingestion of a potentially poisonous substance, it was never proven to be effective in preventing poisoning. Recent research has failed to show benefit for children who were treated with ipecac. This is the key reason for this policy change," the academy said in a statement.

---

In general, survival rates following treatment for major health problems decline as patients age, if for no other reason than that they are more likely to have other health issues. But the key factor is overall health, not merely the patient's birth date. For example, recent research on major heart surgeries indicates that if the total health of a patient is taken into consideration, age alone has little effect on survival rates.

The statistics on heart transplants support that view. A heart transplant recipient in her thirties, like the patient in "Control"

(1-14), has almost a 70 percent chance of being alive five years later. However, the average five-year survival rates for heart transplant recipients in their fifties and early sixties are actually a little bit higher; although statistically the difference is too close to call. Heart transplant recipients sixty-five or older have slightly lower five-year survival rates, but again, the difference is not statistically significant.

So when Dr. House got into a heated argument with the hospital's transplantation committee on behalf of a sixty-five-year-old patient in "Sex Kills" (2-14), the premise of the debate was off the mark. Dr. House lambasted the committee for not valuing his patient simply because of his age. Nonetheless, transplant experts say that while the focus on the patient's age alone was an oversimplification of the process, in some ways the scene did ring true, because the shortage of donated organs forces them to make anguishing choices about who will get a transplant and who won't. Because Dr. House's sixty-five-year-old patient in "Sex Kills" appeared to be in excellent health, except for the bacterial infection that damaged his heart, he might well have been considered a very good candidate for transplantation.

Once a patient is determined to be a good candidate for a transplant, age is not one of the basic criteria used to allocate the organs that become available. The number-one factor is whether a recipient is already so sick that he or she is relying on a machine (such as a left ventricular assist device) to take over some or all of the work of the diseased heart. The next critical factor is how close the recipient is to the donor. The quicker the transfer, the better; a donated heart can't survive outside the body for more than about four hours.

The plot of this episode took a twist when it turned out nobody wanted the heart of a car crash victim at Princeton-Plainsboro Teaching Hospital because test results indicated she was infected with incurable hepatitis C. So Dr. House set out to prove that the test results were wrong. He argued that the brain-dead crash victim probably had another type of infection, one that he could cure; thus making it safe to transplant the woman's heart into his patient.

While the premise of the episode seems typically weird and macabre, that Dr. House would have to "cure" a dead woman in order to save the life of his patient, in reality this sort of treatment is done all the time. In fact, there are detailed protocols spelled out for the treatment of infectious diseases and other conditions that affect the organs of potential donors. Transplant experts say medically treating potential donors, even after brain death, is a vital strategy for dealing with the terribly inadequate supply of donated organs. One group reviewed the major treatment options in an article titled "Care of the Potential Organ Donor" that appeared in the *New England Journal of Medicine.*

"The care of the donor is essentially the simultaneous care of multiple recipients. Vigilant medical management ensures that the greatest number of organs can be recovered in the best possible condition to provide optimal outcomes for the recipients. Current therapies appear to enhance successful organ procurement," the authors wrote.

The article noted that infections do not necessarily rule out organ donation. Bacterial infections can be treated before the organ is transplanted. What's more, transplant statistics indicate recipients of organs from donors with bacterial infections have just as good a chance for long-term survival as other recipients.

Although bacterial infections can be treated with antibiotics, there is no quick and easy cure for viruses like hepatitis B or C. The recipient of an organ infected with hepatitis is likely to become infected and the infection may not be curable. So that means, as Dr. House stated, that a positive test for hepatitis C would make a donor heart unusable, right? Not necessarily. Hepatitis B or C infection can be managed. A patient might well accept the longer term threat of liver damage from hepatitis as preferable to death from heart failure within a week, which is the fate Dr. House's patient faced.

There are some infections that are considered "absolute contraindications" to organ donation. They include HIV, measles, rabies, a type of virus that can cause blood cell cancer (human T-cell leukemia-lymphoma virus), and some others. One of these viruses would indeed close off transplant options, unless Dr. House could find a unique solution. But considering that the shortage of donor organs means early death for many patients, transplant teams and patients could well step forward to accept organs possibly infected with hepatitis C.

Transplant experts use the term "extended criteria" when they talk about organs that are not perfect, but might still help extend the lives of patients waiting for a transplant. In the calculus of transplants, the organs of a young, healthy person who suddenly suffered fatal injuries, say from a crash or act of violence, could be considered "ideal." But when a tragic incident cuts short the life of an older person who may have some chronic health issues, their organs may still have considerable value. Transplant experts ask individuals and families to always consider organ donation, because the unmet need is so immense.

Even though completely restoring health may be too much to expect after a close brush with death, selecting the best treatment is crucial to giving a patient the best chance. And often, selecting the treatment can be every bit as challenging as making the right diagnosis; there are almost always trade-offs and uncertainties.

For typical patients with typical ailments, physicians can consult volumes of advice and recommendations based on mountains of clinical experience and scientific study. But then "typical" doesn't often describe Dr. House's patients. Frequently, he and his team must blaze a fresh trail; and so they reach out for experimental treatments.

## Experimental Treatment

In "Maternity" (1-04), when a virus is spreading through the neonatal unit, Foreman suggests using an experimental antiviral drug that he says produced positive results in a laboratory test. In "Mob Rules" (1-15), a nasty case of hepatitis C is the enemy. Chase suggests using an experimental drug similar to certain antiretroviral treatments for HIV. He points out that it's being tested in dogs. This time, Foreman is a skeptic, concerned that the drug, which has never been tested in a human, might be lethal.

While experimental drugs are sometimes given to people in emergency situations, skepticism is warranted. Just because a drug is new does not mean it is better. Indeed, the Pharmaceutical Research and Manufacturers of America (PhRMA), a pharmaceutical industry trade group, which is an enthusiastic booster of the benefits of new medicines, notes that of every 10,000 compounds that enter laboratory testing, just one will eventually enter regular clinical use. That's a 99.99 percent failure rate. So it is extremely unlikely, if not impossible, that a drug that is still just in laboratory testing would actually help a patient near death.

Laboratory testing of drugs looks at how the experimental molecule affects some component of a disease. For instance, does it kill or weaken a bacterium or virus when they are mixed together in a lab dish? Does the drug latch onto a key protein that the disease uses, in a way that hints it might block the growth or infectious capability of a microbe? Does it bind to and inactivate a toxic by-product of the disease, thus suggesting it might slow the progression in a patient? These are critical questions, but they look at just a few aspects of a disease or condition. Laboratory testing is unable to predict with any certainty how a new drug will act within the incredibly complex biological processes of a living person.

Even if a drug is the one in 10,000 that will ultimately make it from the lab to market, in the early stages of research no one would know what dose to use in a person or even how to give it. Should it be infused, injected, or swallowed? Will it interact with other medications? How long should treatment continue?

The odds are somewhat better for drugs that show positive results in animal testing, like the potential hepatitis treatment touted by Chase in "Mob Rules." But there is a classic response to news that an experimental drug has cured cancer in rats: "I'll recommend it to all the rats I know with cancer."

Although animal test results are far more informative than laboratory results, there are immense differences between the animals and humans in terms of how their bodies metabolize drugs. For instance, one series of animal tests of a compound that is somewhat related to the kind of hepatitis treatment mentioned in "Mob Rules" showed wide differences in how different species handled the drug. Researchers were looking at bioavailability, which is a measure of how much of the drug actually gets into the blood stream. Bioavailabilities ranged from about 20 percent in rats to four times as high, 70 to 80 percent, in dogs and rhesus monkeys. In other words, even after adjusting doses to take into account the different sizes and weights of the animals, the equivalent dose would deliver four times as much of the drug to dogs and monkeys as it would to rats. If all you have is data from animal studies, and without knowing critical information about bioavailability and other factors, it would be very easy to give either too much or too little of a new drug to a patient.

A now-infamous front-page story in the *New York Times* newspaper in 1998 reported great excitement over tests of a class of drugs that had eliminated tumors in mice. The story featured a quote from a prominent scientist predicting a cure for cancer within two years. However, the first two drugs of the new type, angiostatin and endostatin, which are designed to strangle the blood supply to growing tumors, did not produce immediate or dramatic results when they were eventually given to people with cancer. While researchers continue to study angiostatin, endostatin, and other similar drugs, the disappointing experience has been a strong reminder that failure is far more common than success in the world of experimental treatments.

In "Babies and Bathwater" (1-18), Dr. House said that a drug from this class, known as antiangiogenesis drugs or angiogenesis inhibitors because they interfere with the growth of new blood vessels, triggered complete remissions in 30 percent of cancer patients. However, progress has been elusive in the fight against the small-cell lung cancer that the patient had in that episode. A trial of an angiogenesis inhibitor called bevacizumab did garner a lot of interest in 2005 after a trial, that also used standard chemotherapy, produced a 27 percent response rate in patients with a different type of cancer, known as non-small-cell lung cancer. But on average the patients getting the experimental therapy survived for one year; just two months longer than the patients who were given standard therapy. Two months of additional survival can be important, but it's a long way from a cure.

Beyond interspecies differences in drug metabolism, there are also vital differences in the diseases themselves. Cancer in a dog is very similar to, but not quite the same as, cancer in a person. What's more, the diseases in laboratory animals are often artificial. The cancerous tumors in lab mice may be first grown in a lab dish and then placed into the mice. Also, many of the mice are not "normal," but have been bred specially for research. One of the most famous breeds is called "nude" mice. They are hairless, as the name implies; but the feature that's more interesting to researchers is that these mice lack a thymus and cannot produce T cells. Without this critical component of the immune system, the mice do not reject human-cell tumors, allowing researchers to perform more experiments. Other mice have been bred to spontaneously develop various types of cancer, so that researchers can see what the effects of new treatments might be.

These special lab animals play a central role in medical research, but doctors and patients cannot jump to the conclusion that what's good for a lab rat is good for a person.

If a potential treatment passes through laboratory testing and then animal tests, it still usually faces at least three levels of human clinical trials. Phase I is safety testing. These early trials usually involve just a few dozen volunteers. Sometimes they are people with a disease, but often they are healthy volunteers, since the test is just about safety, not effectiveness. The key question: Will the new treatment cause unreasonable side effects? Although results of Phase I tests are sometimes called "promising" or "encouraging," the studies are not designed to demonstrate whether or not the treatment actually produces any benefits. About two-thirds of experimental treatments pass Phase I human trials.

Phase II trials are designed to see if the experimental treatment actually does what it is supposed to do. Most drugs that reach this stage do not go any further, because they don't live up to the hopes raised by lab and animal testing.

Phase III is usually the big clinical trial that either makes or breaks a new treatment. It may involve thousands of patients at multiple locations who are followed for many months or years. This is where researchers find out whether the benefits of a new drug outweigh the side effects . . . and at what dose. Even though drugs go through years of study before reaching this point, drugs going into Phase III human trials are hardly sure things. In fact, up to three out of four fail.

For the one drug in four that does pass the big test, Phase III clinical testing is typically the last stop before a manufacturer applies for FDA permission to market a new drug; but even huge trials don't reveal everything about new drugs. The experiences of the fen-phen diet drug combination, Vioxx pain medication, and many other drugs show that even when drugs look like winners in trials involving thousands of people, when drugs get out in actual clinical use, the benefits may turn out to be smaller, and the risks greater, than had been expected.

Still, for the sake of argument, let's say there is indeed an experimental drug that might help a desperate patient, but it hasn't been through the long process needed to win approval from the FDA. Could a doctor still use it, if it seemed to be the best hope for the patient?

Foreman said one of his medical school professors was developing chemical warfare antidotes for the military that would be just the thing to rescue the teenage boys who were exposed to potentially lethal doses of pesticides in "Poison" (1-08). He made a call and had a batch sent right over.

Actually, it could happen. Not easy or common, but still possible. The FDA has procedures for the emergency use of experimental treatments, including forms to fill out and submit. But physicians can contact an FDA official any time of the day or night by telephone to get a quick okay, if necessary. And FDA regulations specifically authorize use of experimental drugs in emergency situations when there isn't time to go through the normal channels. In general, the emergency arrangement is a one-time deal. The physicians still need to fill out forms and provide information after the emergency is over. And if they want to use the drug again in other patients, the hospital would have to submit paperwork and either join a clinical trial or set up a formal procedure for giving experimental drugs to patients outside of a trial.

But even if FDA approval isn't a problem, finding out about experimental treatments and then getting supplies can be challenging. New drugs are often closely guarded secrets at pharmaceutical companies. In fact, it is against the law for the FDA to even admit the existence of a new drug unless the manufacturer chooses to publicly release the information. And the FDA is not involved in supplying drugs; that is entirely up to the manufacturer or researchers who own the drug. There may be an extremely limited supply of a new medicine and it may be already fully committed to patients in clinical trials.

Patients interested in new drugs are encouraged to enter clinical trials. The federal government operates a web site, clinicaltrials.gov, that lists many such trials. But getting into a trial does not necessarily mean getting a cure. Some trials use placebo or "sham" pills in order to help prove that any effects are actually due to the drug being tested. While many people say they don't want to be given the placebo, the fact is that in most trials, patients on placebo do as well or better than those who get the new drug. New drugs are called "experimental" for a good reason: they haven't been proven to work . . . and they may produce nasty surprises.

---

## Thalidomide

The "poster child" of drug regulation by the FDA is thalidomide.

In the 1960s the drug was approved in several European nations as a sedative. At first, it seemed to work well with few side effects. But no one had performed the type of thorough human testing expected today, including studies of the potential effects on a developing fetus. The consequences of the research shortcuts were tragic. Some 8,000 babies were born missing limbs or with flippers instead of arms.

Before the terrible toll of birth defects was recognized, thalidomide's manufacturer was pushing for approval to sell it in the United States, too. However, as an FDA article notes, one scientist at the agency insisted that more tests were needed. Frances Kelsey, M.D., Ph.D., was not satisfied with results from animal testing. Then the spike in birth defects appeared in Europe. As it turned out, some adults also suffered serious side effects, including permanent, painful numbing of the hands and feet.

Now thalidomide is back . . . in a way. The very properties that make it so damaging to a developing fetus may be useful against certain diseases. In the late 1990s, the FDA finally approved U.S. sales, but not for the drug's original sedative use. The agency okayed selling thalidomide to treat an inflammatory condition that affects people with leprosy, also known as Hansen's disease. Dr. House ordered up a supply to treat a boy with the disease in "Cursed" (1-13). Cameron was taken aback at first, reacting to the historical stigma of thalidomide and its link to horrible birth defects. But Dr. House pointed out that there was little chance that a twelve-year-old boy could get pregnant.

Thalidomide prescriptions are tightly regulated. There's a "black box" warning . . . a highlighted section of the prescribing information that must be distributed with the drug. It says, in part:

WARNING: SEVERE, LIFE-THREATENING HUMAN BIRTH DEFECTS. IF THALIDOMIDE IS TAKEN DURING PREGNANCY, IT CAN CAUSE SEVERE BIRTH DEFECTS OR DEATH TO AN UNBORN BABY. THALIDOMIDE SHOULD NEVER BE USED BY WOMEN WHO ARE PREGNANT OR WHO COULD BECOME PREGNANT WHILE TAKING THE DRUG. EVEN A SINGLE DOSE (1 CAPSULE [50, 100, or 200 mg]) TAKEN BY A PREGNANT WOMAN DURING HER PREGNANCY CAN CAUSE SEVERE BIRTH DEFECTS.

Thalidomide may also have potential benefits for some patients with macular degeneration and certain sores that afflict some people with AIDS.

One remarkable historical footnote: Dr. Kelsey was not a veteran FDA evaluator when she resisted the manufacturers of thalidomide. She had been with the agency only a short time and thalidomide was the first drug application assigned to her. Her stubborn demand for more study became an FDA legend.

---

In most of the cases on *House, M.D.*, the treatment is almost always straightforward and obvious. If it's an infection, knock it right down with a blast of antibiotics or antivirals. If it's a tumor, cut it out. In "TB or Not TB" (2-04), Dr. House is confirming his suspicion of a tumor in the patient's pancreas in one scene . . . and then in the next scene, the patient is checking out of the hospital, fully recovered.

If it's poisoning or other toxic exposure, remove the source.

---

### Cadmium Pot

In "Sports Medicine" (1-12), the combination of weak, brittle bones, fertility issues, and shrunken testes, as well as kidney damage in a professional baseball player had Dr. House and his team stumped, until he noticed that the patient's wife had trouble smelling things. Suddenly low-level cadmium poisoning, probably from smoking marijuana grown in contaminated soil, jumped to the top of the list of possible diagnoses.

All the puzzle pieces fit. Cadmium is linked to bone loss, kidney problems, shrunken testes, and damaged sense of smell. Marijuana and other plants can draw cadmium from the soil and concentrate it. Inhaling cadmium-laced smoke can deliver the toxic heavy metal into the body.

### "Ouch-ouch"

Bone problems linked to cadmium became obvious when investigators discovered the cause of *"itai-itai"* disease in Japan shortly after World War Two. *Itai-itai* literally means "ouch-ouch." The term refers to the pain suffered by patients whose bones frequently broke and did not heal properly. Patients also suffered kidney degeneration.

Eventually, doctors connected *itai-itai* disease to widespread environmental contamination from cadmium mines in the area. After environmental controls were put into place and the environment cleaned up, the cases of *itai-itai* disease dwindled.

The toxic effects of cadmium are sometimes referred to as an acquired form of Fanconi's syndrome, which is an inherited disorder. Our bones are losing and gaining material throughout our lives. The process involves a delicate balancing act. But the kidneys of patients with Fanconi's syndrome excrete key minerals instead of reabsorbing them into the bloodstream. When calcium and other important minerals are lost from bone faster than they are replaced, bones don't grow properly or they fracture.

Even though researchers made the link between cadmium, environmental contamination, and toxic effects in people half a century ago, the threat has not ended. Researchers have seen bone, kidney, and other problems result from levels of cadmium contamination far lower than those seen in the Japanese experience. For instance, pollution from a smelter in Belgium was linked to reduced bone density, higher rates of bone fractures, and abnormally rapid declines in the height of older men and women. The bone damage seen in the Belgian community is thought to be related to kidney damage caused by the cadmium pollution.

Studies by the Argonne National Laboratory in Argonne, Illinois, suggest that workers in factories may be harmed by extremely low levels of cadmium, levels that are currently legal. The researchers think even small exposures to cadmium can accelerate bone loss. Since bone loss, or osteoporosis, is a common problem for older people, the problems of an older factory worker, or someone who retired from a plant where cadmium was present, may be blamed on age, when they may actually be due in part to cadmium exposure.

Other studies link elevated cadmium levels to smaller testes in men. And there is evidence that cadmium and other heavy metals can damage the olfactory neuroepithelium, thus interfering with the sense of smell. In fact, some researchers say that a significant proportion of cases of damage to the sense of smell that are currently listed as "idiopathic," or unexplained, may be caused by exposure to cadmium or other metals.

You can be damaged by cadmium even if you don't work or live anywhere near cadmium mines, smelters, or other industrial sources of heavy metals. Cadmium is found in cigarette smoke. Tobacco plants pull the toxic metal up out of the soil, and then smoking transfers the poisonous material into the lungs.

Elevated cadmium exposure is one hazard of smoking any brand of cigarettes; but the levels of cadmium, and the resulting risks of bone and kidney damage appear to be higher with black-market cigarettes. Studies in Jamaica, the United Kingdom, and elsewhere have documented higher levels of cadmium in illicit cigarettes. A Jamaican study found cadmium levels in tobacco that were fifty times those found in commercial cigarettes. Researchers said the high levels reflected the known high concentrations of cadmium in the soil of the region.

Of course, Jamaica is also known for its production of marijuana. The risk of cadmium exposure may be higher from marijuana than from tobacco. The *Cannabis sativa* plant appears to be unusually efficient at extracting cadmium from soil. Indeed, marijuana or hemp plants may be useful tools in cleaning up toxic waste sites. For example, in one set of tests in Eastern Europe, environmental scientists found that marijuana plants were better than several other crops at pulling heavy metals, particularly cadmium from contaminated soils.

In actual medical treatment, treatment decisions are not always as clear-cut as they appear on *House, M.D.* Is surgery better than drug treatment? Should treatment be aggressive, despite greater risks of side effects, or conservative, even if it means more uncertainty about whether the problem has been solved? Whether the treatment options are experimental or old standbys, how do physicians make the best choices for their patients? One part of answering that question is to ask another one: What's the evidence?

## Evidence-Based Medicine

The term "evidence-based medicine" often triggers a puzzled response. After all, isn't *all* medicine based on evidence? Surprisingly, the answer is no; much of modern medical practice lacks solid scientific proof. Instead, there may be some strong hints from research studies or maybe a long history of clinical experience to support a particular treatment; or perhaps it just seems logical.

That's not to say any treatment that hasn't withstood the most rigorous randomized controlled clinical trials isn't good medicine. It is often said that if aspirin were introduced today as a new experimental drug, it might not win approval, because of the very real risks of potentially life-threatening bleeding or toxic overdoses, in addition to the danger of Reye's syndrome in children. But aspirin also helps millions of people relieve pain and it can substantially reduce the odds of heart attack deaths in people at high risk.

But there are many examples of treatments that everyone "knew" worked, despite a lack of scientific evidence. A famous review of heart treatments performed in the early 1990s reported that although lidocaine injections were routinely used to prevent dangerous heart fibrillations, there weren't any solid studies to support the practice. The lidocaine treatment is still used, but there is strong debate whether it is preferable to alternatives.

In another case involving well-accepted heart therapy, most physicians believed that a set of drugs proven to control serious heart rhythm abnormalities was helpful also to patients who had just slightly abnormal rhythms. It became common practice to give these heart rhythm drugs to patients who had subtle arrhythmias detectable with heart monitors, even though they weren't feeling any symptoms. Then a large trial involving these asymptomatic patients demonstrated that the patients given the popular drugs encainide and flecainide were actually more likely to die than the patients given placebo pills. One of the researchers who led the trial of these antiarrhythmia drugs said many of his colleagues scoffed at the expensive scientific testing of a treatment they all "knew" worked. The heckling ended when the results showed that, in this case, common sense and routine practice were dead wrong.

The drugs are still used to treat patients with more serious heart arrhythmias, where the balance of risks and benefits tips in favor of treatment.

In one way, the personality of Dr. House fits well with the tenets of evidence-based medicine. While most people tend to rely on the opinions of experts, he shows little respect for authority figures or the advice of experts based solely on their reputations. He would not press ahead with a course of treatment just because a senior physician proclaimed it to be the best choice.

And so it is with evidence-based medicine. "Expert opinion" is considered the lowest form of evidence; not worthless, but something that should be used only when nothing better is available. After all, expert opinion may be just the sum of what a single physician recalls from his or her clinical experience, subject to all the vagaries of memory and normal human biases.

Working up the rungs of evidence, just above expert opinion comes "case reports or series." These are collections of clinical experience. They are useful for recording things that have happened, but they have many weaknesses. For instance, a report from Portugal helped Dr. House crack the case of a woman who contracted African sleeping sickness through sexual transmission in the episode "Fidelity" (1-07). However, such a report provides no information about how often something occurs, or whether the treatment used in one case will necessarily produce the same outcomes in other cases.

Up one more rung sit "observational studies." These are the sorts of studies that often get wide attention when they appear to connect everyday activities with certain risks or benefits. For instance, are coffee drinkers any more or less likely to develop heart problems? Is heavy cell phone use associated with a higher risk of brain tumors? Both of these questions have generated plenty of headlines, but the studies behind the news stories have been generally too weak to provide reliable answers. Among the major weaknesses of observational studies is that they may be thrown off by confounding factors . . . or they may have cause and effect backward.

A confounding factor is something the researchers didn't measure that might be the real culprit. For instance, many early studies of vitamin supplements that seemed to support health benefits did not take into account the fact that many people who took the vitamins also ate healthier diets and exercised more than people who didn't take vitamins. And observational studies have to be very careful about making claims about cause and effect because researchers often don't know which came first. For example, are depressed teenagers more likely to drink alcohol or does drinking alcohol cause depression in adolescents? Observational studies have difficulty sorting out that sort of question.

Now we are up to "randomized controlled trials." These are often called the "gold standard" of medical science, because if they are designed and performed properly, they can overcome many problems with human recall, subjective observations, confounding factors, and other challenges. In good randomized controlled trials, hundreds or even thousands of participants are randomly assigned to get one treatment or another or none at all. The treatments are often given in a way that neither the researchers nor the patients know who is getting what—the so-called double blind design.

Randomized controlled trials can provide definitive answers, but there are limitations. They are often costly. They can usually answer only narrow questions, such as whether one drug is better than another drug for patients with a specific set of symptoms; one trial can't tell us how to prevent heart disease or cancer. And it would be unethical to do clinical trials to answer many important questions. For instance, there is evidence from many observational studies that people who drink a bit of wine or other alcoholic beverages seem to have lower rates of heart disease than people who don't drink alcohol at all. But the question remains: Is there something else different about people who drink alcohol in moderation compared to those who do not drink alcohol at all? A randomized controlled trial could settle the matter, but a robust trial would require assigning some nondrinkers to start drinking—an unthinkable condition.

## Whiskey Cure

In the first episode of the second season, "Acceptance," House took a page from old westerns, pulling out a bottle of whiskey to cure what ailed his patient; in this case, methanol poisoning from drinking copy machine fluid. As House and the patient downed shots, he explained that ethanol, the form of alcohol in beverages, binds to toxic formic acid that is a metabolite of methanol, allowing the body to excrete the poison.

Technically, House's colorful cure can work . . . and the recommended dose of eighty-proof whiskey would be about four standard 1½ ounce shots for a 200-pound patient, enough to make him too drunk to drive. But the "whiskey cure" fits better with a Wild West saloon than a modern hospital, according to poison control experts.

Fomepizole is the front-line therapy for methanol poisoning. Rather than sopping up the toxic by-products, an infusion of fomepizole prevents the body from metabolizing methanol into formaldehyde and formic acid in the first place.

The drug is also used to treat people poisoned by ethylene glycol, which is the main ingredient of automobile antifreeze.

---

What could be even better than a randomized controlled trial? Several such trials.

The top rung in the world of evidence-based medicine is held by what is known as a systematic review of randomized controlled trials. Systematic reviews follow a careful protocol for collecting information from multiple trials and then combining all the results in a way that the final product is even more reliable than the results of the individual trials. The method involves some extremely sophisticated statistical methods, but systematic reviews can reveal the best available picture of the state of the art in a particular area.

Examples of recent systematic reviews include reports that birth control pills do not cause weight gain, and that steroid treatment for head-injury patients actually increases their risk of death.

Getting the word out to physicians and health care institutions about medical evidence is one part of ongoing efforts to avoid what are called "unwarranted variations" in medical care. The term refers to the fact that sometimes a patient with a certain condition gets one type of care, and another time a nearly identical patient is given very different care, without a clear medical rationale. Too often it seems that how you are treated may depend less on what you have than on where you are when you have it.

## The Dartmouth Atlas of Health Care

In order to find out more about the kind of care you are likely to get if you are hospitalized, you might want to consult the *Atlas*. That advice might sound odd at first; after all, isn't a heart attack in Peoria the same as one in Paducah, and a tumor in Tallahassee the same as one in Tempe? In general, yes, the medical conditions are the same; but according to the *Dartmouth Atlas of Health Care*, the type of care provided may be quite variable, for reasons that seem to have little to do with science.

The *Dartmouth Atlas* Project is run by the Center for the Evaluative Clinical Sciences at Dartmouth Medical School in Hanover, New Hampshire. The researchers there comb through databases of health care to get a picture of what doctors do . . . and why.

One of the most consistent—and startling—findings of their work is that where you get care is often more important than what you have. For instance, if you are a woman with early stage breast cancer, the science indicates that a conservative lumpectomy and radiation treatment is just as effective as removing the breast with a mastectomy. However, based on data from the early 1990s, while about half the women in some regions of the country were treated with breast-sparing surgery, in other regions almost all patients underwent mastectomies.

There are, of course, conditions for which treatment is quite consistent. When someone falls and fractures a hip, a trip to the hospital is practically guaranteed. There are relatively minor variations in hip fracture hospitalizations between different regions of the country, and those variations are closely linked to the rates of hip fractures themselves. One strange note: People in the inland south, from North Carolina to New Mexico are more likely to break their hips than people in other parts of the country. The reason is unknown.

But the *Dartmouth Atlas* investigators say the medical response to a forearm fracture is a quite different thing. Although forearm fractures are quite painful and the treatment options seem relatively straightforward, patients in some parts of country are almost twice as likely to be hospitalized as those in other parts of the country, where outpatient treatment in the emergency room or a doctor's office is more common.

The *Dartmouth Atlas* findings indicate that physicians and hospitals have local community cultures and habits; that is, their treatment decisions often are more likely to follow consistent local patterns than they are to adhere to objective and universal standards.

There are three major categories of what the *Dartmouth Atlas* researchers call "unwarranted variation":

1. Underuse of most kinds of effective care

2. Misuse of preference-sensitive care

3. Overuse of supply-sensitive care

An example from the first category, underuse of effective care, is poor compliance with the strong recommendation that every heart attack survivor get a prescription for beta blocker medication. No region in the country scores a perfect 100 percent on that standard. In the "best" regions, 80 percent of heart attack survivors are discharged from the hospital with beta blocker prescriptions. But in other regions, the prescription rate is just 10 percent.

Treatment for early stage breast cancer is an example of the misuse of preference-sensitive care. In this type of situation, there is more than one treatment option, and the science does not overwhelmingly favor one or the other. Ideally, patients would choose which they preferred. However, the Dartmouth analysis indicates that the preference of the physician, not the patient, almost always wins out. It appears that Dr. House is not the only physician who thinks he knows better than patients what they should want.

The third category of unwarranted variation in medical practice refers to the tendencies of physicians and hospitals to stay busy. Rather than being demand-sensitive, that is, doing more procedures when the need goes up and cutting back when the need goes down; health care systems tend always to operate near full capacity. So the more hospital beds that are available, the more likely a patient is to be admitted. The more MRI machines in a community, the more scans will be done.

Of course, providing more health care would be a good thing, if it saved more lives and reduced suffering. Unfortunately, the *Dartmouth Atlas* data and information from many other sources indicates more is not always better when it comes to health care. In fact, more health care may be worse for patients.

Every test, every drug, and every procedure sometimes produces errors or harms patients. So the more that is done, the more errors and harm that occur. Also, when supply goes up, doctors and hospitals work their way down the list of patients. After they've taken care of all the patients in urgent need, they start working on the ones with moderate need, and then the ones with minor needs. For example, doubling the number of cardiologists in a community tends to double the number of office visits to cardiologists, without any clear connection to the number of people with heart disease in the community. And when physicians of any variety start working on patients who don't have as much to gain, because they aren't as sick, while still exposing them to the risks of a test or procedure, the balance may tip the wrong way.

This concern is not just hypothetical. Analyses done by the *Dartmouth Atlas* researchers and others show that as hospital capacity goes up, death rates do not decline as you would hope. In fact, death rates are higher in communities that have more hospital beds available per capita.

There have even been a few studies that tried to test the "intensity" of health care the way a new drug would be studied: with a randomized trial. In one study, patients in one group were assigned to frequent clinic visits, while those in the other group were just telephoned at home. The patients who came into the clinic for face-to-face visits were more likely to be hospitalized and even slightly more likely to die.

In another test, researchers studied patients who were being discharged from nine VA medical centers after treatment for diabetes, chronic obstructive pulmonary disease, or congestive heart failure. The patients were randomly assigned to receive either standard follow-up care or to get intensive primary care. The hope was that more care would help keep the patients at home and prevent another hospital stay. But the opposite happened. The patients getting intensive follow-up were actually more likely to end up back in the hospital than the patients who received less care. Interestingly though, the "intensive" patients reported they were more satisfied with their care.

Of course, more care is indeed better in many circumstances. But the blanket assumption that more is always better just doesn't hold up in health care.

The researchers at the *Dartmouth Atlas* and elsewhere have recommended various strategies for bringing medical practice more into line with the scientific evidence and recommended standards; but the task won't be an easy one, because it challenges long-standing traditions, beliefs, and local medical cultures.

## Maggots and Leeches

There is hardly a treatment with a longer medical tradition than bleeding with leeches, which is experiencing a renaissance, although with a somewhat different purpose than in ancient times. And pouring 10,000 maggots on someone's burned belly may sound like medieval torture, but that's just what Dr. House ordered in "Distractions" (2-12).

An article in the journal *Advances in Skin & Wound Care* points out that maggots have actually played a role in U.S. medicine since early in the twentieth century, when a surgeon named William Baer tried applying the little crawly critters to chronic wounds of some children with osteomyelitis, which is a type of bone infection.

Here's how it works: Maggots feed on dead tissue, so they clean away tissue that's not healing and which may be harboring harmful bacteria. This process is called debridement. When the patient's body fails to clear away dead tissue by itself, debridement may be done surgically, by using bandages that help peel away dead tissue, with enzymes, or with the help of maggots. Maggot secretions also may have beneficial properties.

Maggots are regulated by the FDA as medical devices. There is a commercial supplier in Irvine, California, that ships maggots in sterile containers to physicians throughout the country. The maggots come with package inserts that look much like the technical sheets provided with prescription drugs, listing the proper dosage and administration, indications and contraindications, including a notation that the maggots are considered a "single-use-only" item. Oh, the package insert also warns health care practitioners not to let the maggots wander away.

The maggots used for debridement are the larvae of blow flies. Like house flies, blow flies are among the common types of flies found in many homes. Blow flies have shiny metallic colored bodies, as distinct from the dull black of house flies.

Although the maggots depicted on *House, M.D.* were simply spread across the burn wound of the patient, the instructions for use of medical maggots say they should usually be gathered on a moist sterile gauze, which is then applied as a dressing to the wound. Also, the maggot TV stars were much larger than the ones typically used for wound debridement, which are newly hatched and less than one-eighth of an inch long.

The use of medical maggots may continue to grow in part because of the obesity epidemic. As obesity leads to diabetes, which in turn causes blood vessel and nerve damage, it is likely that more people will develop ulcerations.

These wounds are often difficult to heal. Medical maggots can spare some patients from amputation by helping to clean these persistent wounds.

Leeches are another variety of "creepy crawly" that, like maggots, evoke revulsion, fascination, and growing interest for their medical uses. Leeches, too, are technically medical devices when used for patient care, according to the FDA.

But leeches are entirely different animals. They are related to earthworms. The medicinal leech, *Hirudo medicinalis*, lives by sucking blood. In order to keep the blood flowing, they inject an anticoagulant into the bite. That ability to prevent blood from clotting is what has attracted physicians for centuries.

Leeches and bloodletting are mentioned in some of the earliest medical texts of the ancient Greeks. But the type of bloodletting that was practiced for thousands of years finally fell out of favor about a century ago. Current practice applies the same treatment, but for an entirely different purpose.

Rather than draining blood based on the belief that it was somehow therapeutic, the modern use of leeches is narrowly focused on preventing clotting in order to preserve blood flow. Leeches are most often used in reconstructive surgery.

The anticoagulant that leeches produce, hirudin, is effective for several hours. A few leeches are placed at the site of a tissue graft, thus helping to keep veins open. By adjusting the number of leeches and bites, doctors can maintain a slow, steady blood flow for a few days, until new blood vessels have grown into the grafted tissue.

However, leech treatments do carry some risks. Leeches carry a bacterium in their guts that is essential to their health, but which may infect a patient.

Hirudin, the key ingredient in leech saliva, can now be produced by pharmaceutical companies. Researchers are testing it as an alternative to other anticoagulants. However, the fact that hirudin prevents clotting for many hours, which is the feature that makes leeches attractive to reconstructive surgeons, can present a dangerous risk of uncontrollable bleeding in other situations.

Despite their benefits in controlled medical use, leeches are still an annoyance, or worse, in the wild. For instance, doctors in Pakistan reported an unusual case of anemia so severe that the patient needed a blood transfusion. Eventually, they tracked down the source of the problem: a single leech lodged inside the nose of the patient.

---

# Agency for Healthcare Research and Quality

Among the groups trying to reduce unwarranted variations in care is the Agency for Healthcare Research and Quality (AHRQ), a small part of the giant U.S. Department of Health and Human Services. The people at AHRQ (pronounced "arc") describe the agency's job as sponsoring and conducting "research that provides evidence-based information on health care outcomes; quality; and cost, use, and access."

Basically, the agency tries to figure out what works and what doesn't . . . and then spreads the word. For example, one recent report concluded that when a mammogram or breast exam finds a lump, alternatives to breast biopsies, such as MRI scans, are not yet accurate enough to confidently tell women whether or not they have cancer. Another study sponsored by AHRQ cast doubt on hopes that diets high in omega-3 fatty acids can reduce the risk of cancer.

As part of her job as the director of AHRQ, Carolyn M. Clancy, M.D., tries to steer physicians toward using treatments based on solid science. Sometimes that means encouraging the use of guidelines and discouraging physicians from just following their gut instincts or simply doing things the way they've always done them. But Dr. Clancy doesn't see herself as a stodgy bureaucrat trying to rein in quirky individualists like Dr. House.

"An evidence-based approach to delivering health care is derived from studies of groups of patients," she points out, noting that the patients on *House, M.D.* are not part of typical caseloads. "All patients have unique aspects and idiosyncrasies and all of us, I think, would want a doctor who is taking our unique characteristics into consideration when faced with unusual problems. So House does that brilliantly."

Indeed, Dr. Clancy says that even in a health care system that increasingly tries to gather and apply the best evidence, there is a need for physicians who follow their own initiative in any particular case.

She recalled the advice of a health care quality researcher: "He said, 'No matter what happens in a quality system, you want some people to break the rules when it's appropriate.' The hospital protocol may say you do X, Y, and Z, but you know that something else is going to work for this patient and you want somebody who is going to go to bat for you, particularly for people who have some unusual characteristics or some unusual facet of their illness.

"I think we all want that, and I think systems ought to promote that, when it's appropriate," she says.

But when the science is clear, Dr. Clancy wants it to be used. And one way to do that is to promote the use of recommendations, guidelines, or checklists that can help clinicians apply the results of medical research—knowledge that is not only the product of hard work by researchers but also the fruit of altruistic volunteering by countless patients who have participated in clinical trials and other studies.

"Certainly, doctors, like everyone, would prefer to be completely autonomous; and yet as a group, when confronted with the evidence that their less-than-systematic way of going about their daily practice is having negative effects, they are pretty amenable to changing it," she says.

In the types of rare cases featured on *House, M.D.*, standards and guidelines often do not apply, precisely because they are the odd ones, where physicians are operating in uncharted waters, doing the best they can with incomplete information and little applicable guidance from medical literature.

"The rare diagnosis, the unusual patient is something that continues to excite doctors all the time," Dr. Clancy recognizes. But it is in the everyday routine where most of the toll of medical errors lies.

No one criticizes Dr. House, or a physician in real life, if he does his best with a bizarre case and yet fails to save the patient. There was no uproar in "Histories" (1-10) when the diagnosis of rabies came too late. But Dr. House got into a heap of trouble when colleagues suspected he might have carelessly grabbed a syringe with the wrong dose of epinephrine and almost killed a nun having a severe allergic reaction in "Damned If You Do" (1-05).

It's in the routine slips and the inappropriate care of common conditions where Dr. Clancy and other health care quality experts see the opportunities for the greatest gains.

"You can't lose sight of the fact that an awful lot of what doesn't work in health care is pretty systematic, garden-variety stuff, where we know the right answers and we just haven't figured out a way to make it happen routinely," she says.

In one of the early episodes of *House, M.D.* the patient was being poisoned by medicine he was taking for a bad cough. What were supposed to be little yellow pills of prescription cough medicine turned out to be little yellow pills of gout medicine. Prescription drug mix-ups are just one of the many ways health care professionals can make an error. Another unfortunately common type of error was illustrated in "Control" (1-14), when Chase tested the blood flow in a patient's leg, only to realize later that he had tested the wrong leg. The error was corrected without harm to the patient. But when a surgeon operates on the wrong limb, the consequences may be irreversible. It is now recommended that before a patient is put under anesthesia for a knee operation for instance, he or she watch as someone uses an indelible marking pen to write in bold letters "OPERATE ON THIS LEG" and on the other limb "*NOT THIS LEG.*"

It may seem a bit silly, but it is a simple step that can prevent a terrible error. Indeed, in "Three Stories" (1-21) Dr. House and Stacy were shown writing on his legs before he underwent surgery on his damaged thigh muscle.

---

### Dr. Scrawl

Physicians have a reputation for terrible handwriting. Dr. House, though, actually shows quite legible handwriting when he stands at his whiteboard. Dr. Wilson's scrawl is a different matter. At the beginning of "Daddy's Boy" (2-05), Dr. House was late coming in, so Wilson was at the whiteboard, jotting down the patient's symptoms. Cameron, Chase, and Foreman squinted and turned their heads to try to decipher his scrawl.

When medical orders or prescriptions are scrawled, it's more than an annoyance. The FDA, the American Medical Association, and other groups point to poor handwriting as a serious matter of patient safety. Barbara Getty strongly agrees. She and her colleague Inga Dubay teach seminars for health care professionals across the country titled Rx for Handwriting Success. Getty says that despite the proliferation of computers, we are not yet in an all-electronic world.

"Handwriting is still important. If you go into any office, you'll see that handwriting is so essential. Look around your office at all the little notes. They are written by hand, aren't they?" she points out. "My plea to elementary schoolteachers: 'Please teach handwriting.' They think they don't have enough time or are afraid to, but it's not that difficult."

In their seminar and a companion writing manual, Getty and Dubay teach a style of italic handwriting intended to emphasize legibility. It dispenses with the familiar loops of cursive handwriting many of us were taught as schoolchildren.

"If you eliminate the loops in your handwriting," she told one classroom full of doctors, "it may not be gorgeous, but it may be much more legible."

Getty hopes that by cleaning up the scrawls of medical professionals, they are making a difference behind the scenes to improve patient safety.

Of course, many health care institutions have pushed forward with computerized systems in part to try to eliminate errors caused by misunderstood handwriting. Once medical orders are entered into a computer, handwriting is no longer a concern; but as anyone who uses a computer knows, the machines produce their own novel concerns.

A study that went looking for problems associated with a popular computerized physician order entry system found almost two dozen ways the system could create medication error risks. Among the problems: It was sometimes hard to see the complete list of a patient's prescriptions; staffers using the system sometimes mistakenly thought it contained all the important information when actually there were still some paper records with critical notes; the way the computer screens were set up sometimes allowed prescriptions to be entered twice or permitted physicians to enter conflicting prescriptions without realizing it.

The researchers and other commentators said that rather than just looking at the problems that computerized systems might solve, like sloppy handwriting, attention and research should also be directed to the new problems that can crop up when old ways are replaced by high-tech.

---

Medical errors of all types, entirely human as well as computer-assisted, happen far too often.

## To Err Is Human

In 2000, the prestigious Institute of Medicine grabbed the public's attention with a report highlighting the toll of medical errors. The report, *To Err Is Human: Building a Safer Health System*, said that by extrapolating the results of local studies to the entire nation, it appears that between 44,000 and 98,000 Americans die each year as a result of medical errors.

"Even when using the lower estimate, deaths due to medical errors exceed the number attributable to the eighth-leading cause of death. More people die in a given year as a result of medical errors than from motor vehicle accidents (43,458), breast cancer (42,297), or AIDS (16,516)," the report said.

The Institute of Medicine authors emphasized that although

physicians and other health care professionals are, of course, involved in medical errors, they are also essential to solutions.

"The committee believes that a major force for improving patient safety is the intrinsic motivation of health care providers, shaped by professional ethics, norms, and expectations."

When Chase failed to catch a warning sign of a deadly problem in "The Mistake" (2-08), a review committee put all the blame for the death of his patient on his error. Experts in health care quality improvement generally have a different view of the causes of, and solutions for, most medical errors, looking more broadly at chains of events or practice environments, rather than just one error by one individual.

Many of the Institute of Medicine committee's recommendations focused on the need to improve systems of health care. The report suggested improving the reporting of errors, and using oversight groups, protocols and other systemic approaches to reduce the harm that, not surprisingly, sometimes occurs when fallible humans are providing medical care that is often staggeringly complex.

Another Institute of Medicine report, issued the following year, pushed forward with the task of recommending broad changes to the way health care is provided.

> Safety flaws are unacceptably common, but the effective remedy is not to browbeat the health care workforce by asking them to try harder to give safe care. Members of the health care workforce are already trying hard to do their jobs well. In fact, the courage, hard work, and commitment of doctors, nurses, and others in health care are today the only real means we have of stemming the flood of errors that are latent in our health care systems. Health care has safety and quality problems because it relies on outmoded systems of work.
>
> —*Crossing the Quality Chasm: A New Health System for the 21st Century* (2001)

Dr. House might well bristle at further encroachment on his freedom to practice medicine as he sees fit, but the days of the solo practitioner who could master and competently practice medicine unfettered are long gone, if they ever existed.

## Outcomes

One mantra of efforts to improve the quality of health care quality is "outcomes, outcomes, outcomes." What are the results for patients? Do they die or do they live? And if they live, how well?

Dr. House is focused on the crisis at hand. References to what happens to patients later are minimal at best. Sometimes, like the pregnant woman with lung cancer in "Babies and Bathwater" (1-18) or the young college graduate with radiation poisoning in "Daddy's Boy" (2-05), they die. Sometimes, like the heavy-set ten-year-old girl who suffered a heart attack in "Heavy" (1-16) and then was successfully treated for Cushing's disease, they depart the hospital better than ever. Occasionally, as in "Hunting" (2-07), the immediate mystery, in this case liver cysts, is solved, but the patient still has big problems; this patient was left to continue fighting HIV/AIDS.

But the general impression at the end of the episode is that the patients live happily ever after, like the heart transplant recipient in "Control" (1-14) whose surgeon pronounced, "She'll outlive us all."

The most common outcome for real-world patients is somewhere in the middle; a crisis averted usually leaves important health issues to manage. A look at one of the dramatic accomplishments of modern medicine is instructive.

Between 1950 and the end of the twentieth century, heart disease death rates plummeted by more than half, when the aging of the population is taken into account. Of course, everyone dies of something eventually, but the chances of dying of heart disease at any particular age are much lower now than in decades past, so a fifty-year-old man today is much less likely to die of heart disease than a fifty-year-old man was back in 1950. There are many reasons for the improvement. The fact that fewer people smoke is probably the biggest reason. Diet and physical activity play roles, too. But medicine can take its share of credit. In terms of prevention, treatment for high blood pressure and high cholesterol help delay the progression of heart disease.

If you do suffer a heart attack or sudden cardiac arrest today, the medical system is more prepared than ever before. Automated external defibrillators, firefighters, police and other first responders trained to provide some immediate medical assistance, Advanced Life Support ambulances, and other factors mean patients can have their hearts shocked back to normal rhythms on the spot, without waiting to get to a hospital. Clot-busting medicines and emergency angioplasty treatments can clear away blockages and restore blood flow to the muscle of the heart quickly, thus preventing much of the damage of a heart attack. Many more people today return to normal life shortly after a heart attack.

But these heart attack survivors are not cured.

The underlying disease process that led to the heart attack is still there, even after the heart attack itself is over. A heart attack or other major health crisis typically transforms a person into a patient permanently. Doctor visits, prescriptions, lifestyle modification programs all become part of the individual's new routine.

People who have had serious heart attacks have an increased risk of developing heart failure, which means their hearts cannot pump blood as effectively as they should. So although they've been saved from one threat, they remain vulnerable. Even as medicine rescues more people from heart attacks, the number of hospitalizations for congestive heart failure in the United States has doubled in the last fifteen years to about a million hospital admissions a year. Even those heart failure patients who manage to stay out of the hospital often have to take piles of pills and keep up with frequent clinic visits to manage the condition.

Progress against cancer also raises new issues. The good news is that the age-adjusted death toll of cancer in the United States is dropping. As with heart disease, antismoking efforts deserve the biggest round of applause. But treatments have also improved, especially for certain childhood cancers.

About one million Americans develop cancer each year, not including common minor skin lesions. At the same time, the number of cancer survivors is growing. More than 10 million Americans have been hit with a diagnosis of cancer and survived the immediate crisis. However, in many cases the word "cured" might paint too rosy a picture. Cancer survivors often carry a burden of aftereffects from the disease and treatment. They usually remain at an increased risk of developing cancer again, and thus need more intense follow-up monitoring.

Success against cancer is typically measured by looking at the proportion of patients who are still alive five years after being diagnosed. The five-year survival rate is a useful yardstick, but it also has weaknesses. The most important factor that determines five-year survival rate is not the treatment, but the type of cancer. Very few patients diagnosed with lung cancer are still alive five years later, in part because the disease is usually far along and moving quickly when it is discovered. On the other hand, almost all men found to have prostate cancer live at least five more years, mostly because prostate cancers usually grow very slowly.

It is important to distinguish between overall survival, disease-free survival, and progression-free survival. Overall survival counts everyone who is still kicking, no matter how sick. Disease-free survival is closer to what most people think of when they hear the word "cure"; it counts only those patients who have no detectable traces of cancer. Progression-free survival is a term that is growing in significance; it counts the patients whose cancers have not gotten any worse than they were at the start of the measuring period. As more cases of cancer are held in check by treatments, rather than completely eradicated, progression-free survival will become a more common standard. It signifies part of the shift from thinking about cancer as an acute crisis to looking at it as a chronic disease that people can live with for years or even decades.

One notable pitfall of using five-year survival as a measure of success is the peculiar effect of "lead-time bias." When mammography became routine, five-year survival rates for breast cancer rose. The same thing happened after the introduction of the PSA blood test for prostate cancer. In both cases, the main reason for the jump in five-year survival was not that patients were necessarily dying any later, but because their tumors were being found earlier, thus starting the five-year countdown sooner. Early detection may indeed help people live longer, but it can also just mean that they get the bad news about cancer sooner, and then spend more years as a patient, without significantly altering the dates of their deaths. The oft-heard claim that early detection is critical to improving cancer survival should be examined with at least some skepticism; because it is true only when treatment actually helps patients live beyond the dates they probably would have died if the cancer had not been detected early, rather than merely boosting five-year survival statistics by moving the starting gates.

These two brief examples of heart disease and cancer reflect a broad trend. We are living through a major health transition. Sudden crises of the type depicted on *House, M.D.* are dwindling. Medicine is shifting its focus away from responding to acute episodes and realigning toward ongoing management of chronic conditions. We are living longer, but increasingly we are living with some health issues, ranging from a touch of arthritis or an elevated cholesterol level to heart failure or diabetes.

## Life and Death

Dr. House is fond of pointing out that if the team makes the wrong diagnosis or gives the wrong treatment, the patient dies. Well, ultimately everyone dies; but in general we are doing it later and later.

At the dawn of the twentieth century, a baby born in the United States could expect to live about forty-seven years on average. A baby born at the start of this millennium can expect, on average again, to live about seventy-seven years. That's an additional three decades of life expectancy.

However, those figures can be misleading. It is not the case that a century ago, the obituary columns were filled with the names of people who had died in their late forties. Childhood deaths, often from infectious diseases, were routine. In 1900, one out of every three deaths was that of a child younger than five years old. The many lives that were exceedingly brief thus pulled down the average life expectancy. In 1997, children under five accounted for just one out of every seventy deaths.

But how much credit do doctors and medicine get for the thirty-year increase in average life expectancy at birth? The development of the polio vaccine in the 1950s was perhaps the biggest blockbuster medical story of the century, but the dramatic decline in childhood deaths from infectious diseases began well before that landmark event. Indeed, by 1950 life expectancy at birth had already jumped to sixty-eight years, more than two-thirds of the total increase during the twentieth century. Cleaner water, more and better food, better housing, and other improvements in living and social conditions provided healthy benefits. Working toilets and good public health departments and better social and living conditions prevent many more early deaths than an army of Dr. House clones could ever hope to. After taking all those factors into account, many estimates credit medicine with providing perhaps five years, or only about one-sixth, of the increase in life expectancy at birth that occurred during the last century.

Life expectancy at birth is not the only way to measure things. It's also important to look at the other end of life . . . our senior years, when things are wearing down and we turn to health care more frequently. An average American who turned sixty-five in 1950 could look forward to about fourteen more years of life. In 2000, the average sixty-five-year-old American has a life expectancy of eighteen years. That's an increase of just four years during the last half century.

Meanwhile, what we are paying for health care is rocketing up. In 1960, the per capita spending on health care was less than $150. In 2000, health care spending per person was more than $4,600. The projections for the next decade are staggering. By 2015, national health expenditures are predicted to almost double to a total tab of about $4 trillion a year. That means that when you look at everything produced in the nation, the gross domestic product, from cars to food to entertainment to housing to education and so on, 20 percent of all economic production, or one dollar in five, will involve health care.

Some of the increase has to do with the graying of the nation; but not as much as many people think. A big reason that health care spending is shooting up is all the new medicines and devices that physicians like Dr. House can employ in their personal battles against disease and death.

The MRI and CT scanners that Dr. House and his team throw at every medical question. The exotic new drugs that they scramble to get for their patients. It all costs money and we all pay a share . . . even if we never have a serious illness. About 70 percent of health care spending is consumed on behalf of just 10 percent of the people in the country.

Discoveries and experiments that have come out of the National Institutes of Health (NIH) over the last several decades have helped fuel the enormous growth of both medical knowledge and medical technology, including the science behind many of the drugs and devices available to hospital physicians. Elias Zerhouni, M.D., the director of the NIH, is one of the leading proponents of biomedical research. But in a recent interview with Barbara Culliton, a deputy editor of the journal *Health Affairs*, he said the direction of medical research must change.[1]

"If you looked at the medical team caring for one patient in 1960, you probably had the doctor and nurse and part-time work from a laboratory person—two and half people. Today, to render the care we're rendering, you're talking about seventeen, eighteen, or nineteen people per patient per encounter. Today, a patient is likely to get services from radiology and pathology, plus an internist or other specialist, and drugs, plus administration, billing, and things like that. Health care has become, if you will, an activity that has grown to a sort of mass customization, with many tests and consultations," Dr. Zerhouni told the journal interviewer.

"The most expensive way to practice medicine is to do it the way we do it, where every interaction can involve as many as twenty people. So the transaction costs are enormous. My view is that we are going to have to make major changes, not changes at the margins," he added.

"If you want to transform medicine, it has to be from something other than the curative paradigm: Wait until you're sick and then come and see me, and I'll do what I can. That has been true for 5,000 years. Now we have to do something different."

Dr. Zerhouni says we should look beyond merely treating illness, beyond even preventing illness, in order to try preemptive action against the fundamental dysfunctions within our bodies that eventually lead to illness. He admits that researchers are only beginning to glimpse how such preemptive medicine might work. But Dr. Zerhouni

1. From "Extracting Knowledge from Science: A Conversation with Elias Zerhouni," Barbara J. Culliton, *Health Affairs*, published online March 9, 2006, www.healthaffairs.org.

says medicine cannot simply continue doing more of what it does so much of now, that is, more of the type of intense and desperate battle against advanced disease that is Dr. House's specialty.

"If we keep practicing the medicine we know today the same way for twenty-five years, we will have lost the game," Dr. Zerhouni told *Health Affairs*.

## A Global View

So far we've been reviewing the statistics for just the United States. Things are both similar and very different in other nations. The cost of health care is rising in every developed nation. But the United States has a big lead, spending more than twice as much per person as other leading industrialized nations. Unfortunately we don't seem to be getting a longevity bonus for that extra investment. The United States has been steadily slipping down the rankings of national life expectancy. We are now lagging behind dozens of other nations . . . and the United States is just barely ahead of Mexico.

Still, even if the high-tech medical model hasn't produced a health utopia, if you were struck down by a medical mystery, wouldn't you want to have someone like Dr. House training the full strength of his diagnostic and treatment armamentarium on your case? Let's take a look at what it might be like to be his patient.

# SEVEN

# Bedside Manner

**D**r. House's strength is his diagnostic skill . . . not his communication skills or ability to work with the team. He definitely is not kept around because he's fun to work with, or for his bedside manner. Indeed, Dr. House tries to avoid being at the bedside if at all possible.

The patient in the first episode put her finger on his antisocial attitude and connected it to the chronic pain and disability from his damaged leg.

"So you hide in your office, refuse to see patients because you don't like the way people look at you. You feel cheated by life so now you're gonna get even with the world," the patient says after Dr. House finally comes in to see her.

When generous donor and short-lived chairman of the board Edward Vogler presses Dr. Cuddy to explain why she keeps Dr. House on the staff, she defends his skill, not his personal appeal.

"He makes you miserable. Eight years he's worked here, never made a dime for you, never listened to you," Vogler says in "Mob Rules" (1-15).

"He can change," Cuddy replies.

"He hasn't changed in eight years. Either he can't change, or you can't change him. You have no idea how many times he's lied to you, undercut your authority, made you look like crap to other doctors."

"Yes, I hate him, and here I am, desperately trying to protect his job."

Technical skill is of paramount importance when tackling difficult medical cases. But physicians are supposed to be healers, not just mechanics who happen to work on human bodies.

The editors of a leading medical textbook, *Harrison's Principles of Internal Medicine*, 16th edition, quote their predecessors who edited the first edition:

"No greater opportunity, responsibility, or obligation can fall to the lot of a human being than to become a physician. In the care of the suffering, [the physician] needs technical skill, scientific knowledge, and human understanding . . . Tact, sympathy, and understanding are expected of the physician, for the patient is no mere collection of symptoms, signs, disordered functions, damaged organs, and disturbed emotions. [The patient] is human, fearful, and hopeful, seeking relief, help, and reassurance."

Dr. House seems to have little interest in anything beyond the collections of symptoms and signs his patients bring to the hospital.

The current editors state that physicians should be confident, but not arrogant. Dr. House seems to have trouble staying on the right side of the line dividing the two attributes.

A survey published in the *Journal of Family Practice* in 2001 that looked at what makes patients trust their physicians found that caring and comfort are as important as technical competency. Communication skills, both in terms of what physicians say and how good they are at listening, also are strongly related to patient satisfaction, according to this survey.

## Breaking Bad News

The communication skills of physicians are put to the test when they must deliver bad news to a patient. Delivering the diagnosis of a life-threatening illness, or telling a patient that treatment is unlikely to succeed, is difficult for doctors. And it is something that they are often ill prepared to do.

When it looks like treatment for radiation poisoning will fail near the end of "Daddy's Boy" (2-05), Wilson tiptoes around the bleak prognosis. He tells the patient's father that his son probably won't be able to fight off infections spreading through his body. Wilson never says in plain language that the young man is dying. We don't see whether any of the physicians ever deliver the bad news to the patient. Instead, the last word in this episode is the father's, as he falsely tells his son that he's going to be fine.

In the first episode of the second season, "Acceptance" (2-01), Cameron spends most of the show trying to disprove the existence of a lung cancer that, deep down, she knows will kill her patient. Wilson and House both urge Cameron to tell her patient the truth, but she resists. She doesn't even tell the patient that lung cancer is a possibility as long as there is a shred of a chance of some other diagnosis.

In real life, breaking bad news to patients isn't any easier. Medical school and other training are almost entirely focused on cure and management of illnesses. Death is not only bad news for the patient; many physicians also feel a sense of personal failure. One of the leading experts in lung cancer says it is hard to recruit young doctors into his field in part because most patients die after a relatively short period.

Only in recent years have some programs begun to train young physicians to deliver bad news. One physician/researcher who has led workshops on delivering bad news to patients says that such practices can help boost the confidence levels of physicians. He says much of the advice involves simple measures, such as making sure to have a comfortable, private setting. "Give them a warning shot," he says. "For example, 'What I am going to tell you is very serious, and I'm very sorry I'm going to have to tell you this information. Is this a good time for us to talk about this?,' so someone can muster their emotional energies and be prepared and not be hit over the head."

Other experts recommend what they term a "patient-centered" communication style, in which the physician is careful to monitor how the patient is receiving the news, to make sure he or she understands what is being said and isn't overwhelmed by hearing too much too fast. After testing three types of communication on students who were imagining how they would feel if they were actually patients hearing bad news, researchers in Zurich, Switzerland, reported that patient-centered communication got the best response. They said that patients tend not to respond as well to blunt statements that just lay out the medical facts without considering the patient's feelings. Also, an overly emotional delivery that focuses on just how sad the news is also has drawbacks.

"Research has shown that if bad news is communicated badly it can cause confusion, long-lasting distress, and resentment; if done well, it can assist understanding, acceptance, and adjustment," Professor Lesley Fallowfield, D.Phil., and Valerie Jenkins, D.Phil., at the University of Sussex, England, wrote in an article reviewing research on how physicians deliver bad news to patients.

Good communication with patients is a key part of providing good care, but it may also serve the physician's interests. There's an old saying: "Nice docs don't get sued."

In a report on malpractice and patient complaints in the *Journal of the American Medical Association*, Gerald Hickson M.D. and his colleagues commented that "Patients who saw physicians with the highest numbers of lawsuits were more likely to complain that their physicians would not listen or return telephone calls, were rude, and did not show respect."

Sounds like a description of Dr. House in a way, doesn't it?

At the close of "Poison" (1-08), the mother of a patient is pushing her son in a wheelchair toward the exit when they passed Dr. House and Foreman. The son had been unconscious for most of the episode.

"Who are they?" the boy asks. "Oh, they're the arrogant jerks that saved your life," she replies.

Knowing that Dr. House was an arrogant jerk when she hired him, Dr. Cuddy said she had set aside $50,000 a year for legal expenses. However, she must have been just talking about routine legal work, not payments for medical malpractice claims, which average several times that much.

It should be noted that although malpractice premiums can be extremely expensive for obstetricians, neurosurgeons, and certain other specialists, and the average size of malpractice payments has been rising along with everything else in medicine, the total cost of malpractice payments is still just a tiny part of health care spending. A recent analysis by economist Amitabh Chandra, Ph.D., and his colleagues that appeared in the journal *Health Affairs* indicates that when you spread all malpractice payments made on behalf of physicians across the population, they probably add only about a dollar a month or just over twelve dollars a year to per capita health care spending.

## Hippocratic Oath

But let's get back to the ideals of medical practice. The most famous statement, of course, is the Hippocratic Oath. But you might be surprised to learn that although the ancient Greek physician Hippocrates did say something like "Do no harm," those words are not in the classical version of the oath itself.

---

## Hippocratic Oath–Classical Version

I swear by Apollo Physician and Asclepius and Hygieia and Panaceia and all the gods and goddesses, making them my witnesses, that I will fulfil according to my ability and judgment this oath and this covenant:

To hold him who has taught me this art as equal to my parents and to live my life in partnership with him, and if he is in need of money to give him a share of mine, and to regard his offspring as equal to my brothers in male lineage and to teach them this art–if they desire to learn it–without fee and covenant; to give a share of precepts and oral instruction and all the other learning to my sons and to the sons of him who has instructed me and to pupils who have signed the covenant and have taken an oath according to the medical law, but no one else.

I will apply dietetic measures for the benefit of the sick according to my ability and judgment; I will keep them from harm and injustice.

I will neither give a deadly drug to anybody who asked for it, nor will I make a suggestion to this effect. Similarly I will not give to a woman an abortive remedy. In purity and holiness I will guard my life and my art.

I will not use the knife, not even on sufferers from stone, but will withdraw in favor of such men as are engaged in this work.

Whatever houses I may visit, I will come for the benefit of the sick, remaining free of all intentional injustice, of all mischief and in particular of sexual relations with both female and male persons, be they free or slaves.

What I may see or hear in the course of the treatment or even outside of the treatment in regard to the life of men, which on no account one must spread abroad, I will keep to myself, holding such things shameful to be spoken about.

If I fulfill this oath and do not violate it, may it be granted to me to enjoy life and art, being honored with fame among all men for all time to come; if I transgress it and swear falsely, may the opposite of all this be my lot.

—Translation from the Greek by Ludwig Edelstein, from *The Hippocratic Oath: Text, Translation, and Interpretation*, by Ludwig Edelstein (Baltimore: Johns Hopkins Press, 1943).

---

Young doctors typically do swear an oath as they graduate from medical school, but there is no standard version. And swearing an oath is a relatively recent practice. Howard Markel, M.D., Ph.D., wrote in the *New England Journal of Medicine* that in 1928 only about one out of five medical schools in North American administered an oath during commencement ceremonies. Now oaths are nearly universal at U.S. medical schools.

For example, the graduating students of the Yale University School of Medicine's Class of 2004 adopted the following modified oath.

---

## A Yale Physician's Oath

Now being admitted to the high calling of the physician, I solemnly pledge to consecrate my life to the care of the sick, the promotion of health, and the service of humanity.

I will practice medicine with conscience and in truth. The health and dignity of my patients will be my first concern. I will hold in confidence all that my patients relate to me. I will not permit considerations of gender, race, religion, sexual orientation, nationality, or social standing to influence my duty to care for those in need of my service.

I will respect the moral right of patients to participate fully in the medical decisions that affect them. I will assist my patients to make choices that coincide with their own values and beliefs.

I will try to increase my competence constantly and respect those who teach and those who broaden our knowledge by research. I will try to prevent, as well as cure, disease.

When I am qualified to instruct, I will impart my knowledge gladly, hold my students and colleagues in affectionate esteem, and encourage mutual critical evaluation of our work.

In the spirit of those who have inspired and taught me, I will seek constantly to grow in knowledge, understanding, and skill and will work with my colleagues to promote all that is worthy in the ancient and honorable profession of medicine. I will maintain the honor and the noble traditions of the medical profession. My behavior will be honorable and thoughtful and reflect justice toward all.

If I fulfill this Oath and do not violate it, may it be granted to me to enjoy life and the practice of the Art. This pledge I make freely and upon my honor. May my faith strengthen my resolve.

—Yale University School of Medicine Commencement 2004

---

In 2002 a group of medical societies and foundations in the United States and Europe published what they call a "Physician Charter." The authors said the statement is designed to meet the challenges of medical practice in the new millennium.

The charter is founded on three principles:

*Principle of primacy of patient welfare.* This principle is based on a dedication to serving the interest of the patient. Altruism contributes to the trust that is central to the physician-patient relationship. Market forces, societal pressures, and administrative exigencies must not compromise this principle.

*Principle of patient autonomy.* Physicians must have respect for patient autonomy. Physicians must be honest with their patients and empower them to make informed decisions about their treatment. Patients' decisions about their care must be paramount, as long as those decisions are in keeping with ethical practice and do not lead to demands for inappropriate care.

*Principle of social justice.* The medical profession must promote justice in the health care system, including the fair distribution of health care resources. Physicians should work actively to eliminate discrimination in health care, whether based on race, gender, socio-economic status, ethnicity, religion, or any other social category.

—"Medical Professionalism in the New Millennium: A Physician Charter," a project of the ABIM Foundation, ACP-ASIM Foundation, and the European Federation of Internal Medicine as published in *Annals of Internal Medicine*, February 5, 2002

Dr. House does appear to put patient welfare first, regardless of market forces or social pressures, and he certainly has only contempt for administrative exigencies.

In "Acceptance" (2-01), he fights to find a cure for a condemned murderer, despite Foreman's doubts about whether the patient is worth the effort. Dr. House peppers Foreman with questions about how doctors should decide which patients are worthy of which treatments. He asks whether a child molester would deserve to get antibiotics but not MRIs; thus showing how quickly physicians would be sucked into a moral quicksand, if they tried to judge the "worth" of their patients.

## Physicians and Executions

Physicians are often in attendance at the executions of condemned prisoners in the United States. But the American Medical Association takes a dim view of physician's facilitating capital punishment.

According to the association's policies on medical ethics, physicians should not participate in executions in any official capacity. They may provide tranquilizers to relieve the prisoner's anxiety, but only if the prisoner makes the request.

The AMA policy says physicians should not even declare a prisoner dead. Why not? In part, because the method of execution may not work the first time. Then the physician could be drawn into determining whether and how the execution should proceed. According to news reports, in 1984 a prisoner in the electric chair in Georgia did not die right away. He was left struggling for breath while the executioners prepared to deliver another shock. After two physicians determined the prisoner was still alive, he was electrocuted. Georgia has since switched to lethal injection.

Also, according to the AMA, when there are questions about the legal competence of a prisoner, a physician should not be the one to make the determination, although he or she may offer a medical opinion as part of the legal process. If a prisoner is declared legally incompetent, physicians are not supposed to provide treatment to restore competency, unless the death sentence is commuted before treatment begins.

Similar opposition to the participation of physicians and other health care professionals in capital punishment comes from the American College of Physicians, the American Public Health Association, and other groups.

The policies of these organizations are not mandatory. Physicians are not unanimous in their views of capital punishment and some do participate in the process.

Dr. House's disdain for administrative rules and restrictions seems boundless. In the episode "Hunting" (2-07), the fact that a request to perform a difficult test creates administrative hassles seems to make Dr. House more, not less, inclined to do it. When Cameron suggests the test, Dr. House practically giggles as he contemplates the paperwork that Cuddy will need signed.

The principle of social justice also fits well with Dr. House's world view. In "Histories" (1-10), Foreman is leery about a homeless woman brought in after she collapsed during a police raid. But House jumps right into the case with the same fervor he would show when tracking the source of a wealthy donor's pain. Actually, much greater fervor.

In "Cursed" (1-13), a boy has pain and problems breathing that sound like garden-variety pneumonia to Dr. House. Cuddy persists at getting him to take an interest in the case . . . and he smells the influence of wealth.

"The way you're ignoring my question . . . wow, they're extremely big donors!" House scoffs.

But what about the principle of patient autonomy? Well, two out of three ain't bad. When it comes to violating the right of patients to decide what they want to do, even if it is not what he recommends, Dr. House has a rap sheet a mile long.

During a flashback scene in "Three Stories" (1-21), Dr. House and Stacy are arguing about the best treatment for his damaged leg.

"If this were any other patient, what would you tell them to do?" Stacy asks.

"I would say it's their choice," Dr. House replies.

"What! Not a chance! You'd browbeat them until they made the choice you knew was right."

## Dr. Schwarzenegger-Welby

"He is a kind of Dr. Schwarzenegger-Welby. He's armed with all the weapons, but he's a solo practitioner from 1955." That's how bioethicist Arthur Caplan, Ph.D., describes the way Dr. House blasts away at diseases with all the latest drugs and devices of modern medicine, while eagerly disregarding the constraints of regulations and bureaucracy, and at the same time echoing the private solo practitioner of decades gone by.

Of course, House displays compassion only grudgingly. His version of the old Dr. Marcus Welby has all the focus on the single patient in front of him, but without the warm and fuzzy aura that surrounded that actor who played a doctor on TV for an earlier generation.

As the director of the Center for Bioethics at the University of Pennsylvania in Philadelphia, Dr. Caplan is well versed in the obligations and responsibilities that physicians have to their patients and to their colleagues. His assessment of House's meager social skills and frequent disregard of the feelings and desires of others is blunt.

"Such a physician would have a very short career," he says. "He would be too busy defending himself in court to spend any time practicing medicine, because he would be rightly accused of lying, not charting things, going against direct requests of competent patients, and also not practicing consistent with accepted medical standards.

"House is some kind of iconoclastic solo guy who can do it all. But there isn't any such person. He'd be viewed by his peers as an intolerable, obnoxious dolt. You have to have social skills to work in modern medicine."

House routinely violates patient directives. In the episode "DNR" (1-09) he saves a patient who had signed a DNR, a "do not resuscitate" order, and then dismisses the objections of his colleagues, declaring he wants to practice medicine, rather than debate ethical questions. However, ethics and medicine are inseparable. The goal of medicine is not simply to keep hearts beating and lungs pumping as long as possible; it is to serve the interests of the patient.

Dr. Caplan underscores that the disease is the patient's disease, not the doctor's. And in the real world, patients frequently do not recover; they do not often face simple and clear-cut choices between life and death. The regular challenge for a physician is to assist the patient with managing an illness and ultimately the manner of death using ways and means that are consistent with the patient's values.

But doesn't success excuse much of House's behavior . . . and don't we admire the nimble and effective way he knifes through red tape and meddling bureaucrats? Don't we wish our health care world were more like the version on *House M.D.*?

"No. We'd hate it," says Dr. Caplan. "You would have reinvented medicine circa 1960. And people didn't like it. They felt talked down to. They felt bullied. They felt left out of crucial decisions."

Dr. Caplan concedes that if a doctor did have House's nearly perfect record of correct diagnoses and seemingly miraculous cures, then he might get away with boorish behavior, sloppy dress, and insubordination. But no such doctor exists. In the real world, physicians are fallible, treatment options are often less then ideal, and dramatic cures are few and far between.

There are powerful reasons medicine has left behind the era in which independent physicians were unquestioned masters of their realms.

"Would people like it if there were less bureaucracy, red tape, and fewer lawyers? Yes. But they really wouldn't want a world in which the doctor makes every decision and basically blows off the patient and blows off his colleagues. Medicine today is practiced in teams and it takes a lot of cooperation to deliver health care," Dr. Caplan says.

Patients do want their physicians to recommend which testing or treatment options seem to be the best. And many patients want their physicians to call the shots. Medical expertise is what they are paying for, after all. But while science and clinical experience are necessary components of the decision-making process, they are not the whole story.

When a woman suffering chest pain from heart disease has to decide between taking pills that can ease the condition or undergoing cardiac bypass surgery that can make her feel better and improve her daily life, the patient is the only one who can merge the medical facts with her personal values and beliefs, in order to decide whether the potential additional rewards of surgery outweigh the risks of complications or even death.

When a man is told he has prostate cancer and that surgery or radiation can reduce the odds the cancer will spread, but that doctors cannot confidently promise he will actually have a longer life as a result—and that the treatment is likely to leave him impotent and perhaps needing to wear a diaper—physicians should not impose their beliefs about the relative values of quality and quantity of life.

Unfortunately, patients may not be given even basic information with which to make an informed decision. According to a study in the *Annals of Internal Medicine* published in 2004, less than 10 percent of the educational materials provided to prostate cancer patients described all the treatment options. And even when materials did at least mention all the options, they did not provide comprehensive information about the risks and benefits of each treatment. Each year in the United States, almost a quarter million men have to decide what to do after being hit with a prostate cancer diagnosis. It seems very few are given adequate tools to exercise their right to make informed medical decisions.

## Informed Consent

Rather than simply agreeing to whatever a physician recommends, patients are supposed to provide informed consent, meaning that not only do they agree with the decision, they understand what they are agreeing to. If challenged later, physicians are not supposed to be able to get away with the excuse that, "The poor sap signed the form; it's not my fault he didn't understand the fine print!" Too bad that standard isn't required of loan agreements and computer software installations.

According to a statement from the American Medical Association, the communication process that leads to informed consent for a medical procedure is not just an ethical ideal; it is required by law in every state. Although informed consent has a long history in medical ethics, the legal history is only about fifty years old.

Physicians generally do want patients to understand their medical options, but effectively communicating the necessary information can be challenging.

In "Paternity" (1-02), Foreman tried to talk to the patient's parents about a treatment option; but then he gave up.

"So we've confirmed that the problem is this mutated virus," Foreman says near the end of the episode. "The treatment for SSPE is intraventricular interferon. We implant an Ommaya reservoir under the scalp, which is connected to a ventricular catheter that delivers the antiviral directly to the left hemisphere."

"You want us to consent to this? I don't even understand what you're talking about," the patient's father replies.

"Well, the antiviral . . . Look, I'm sorry, I can explain this as best I can, but the notion that you're going to fully understand your son's treatment and make an informed decision, is, is kind of insane," Foreman says. "Now here's what you need to know: It's dangerous, it could kill him, you should do it."

In this case, Foreman seems to quit before even trying. Many doctors obtain informed consent for the use of Ommaya reservoirs to deliver drugs directly to a patient's brain. Here's an example of an excerpt from a consent form for a cancer therapy trial:

---

### Surgical Procedure

Two to six weeks after the completion of radiation therapy you will undergo a surgical procedure to place a special type of catheter or tube, called a modified Ommaya reservoir, into the middle of the tumor location in your brain. The only part of the catheter that you will be able to see or feel will be under the skin of your scalp.

## Risks Associated with Ommaya Reservoir

Infection

Membrane rupture, which would result in replacement of the reservoir

---

And the drug, interferon, is routinely used to treat hepatitis and other diseases. Introducing the drug directly into spaces in the brain, known as ventricles, is a bit unusual, but this intraventricular treatment does not seem to be an extraordinarily complex situation.

The fatalistic attitude about informed consent displayed by Foreman in this episode of *House, M.D.* appears to have been "created to have some considerable shock value . . . at least I hope that this is the case and that no one would treat their patients like this," says Craig Campbell, M.D. Dr. Campbell is a pediatric neurologist at the Children's Hospital of Western Ontario and the University of Western Ontario in London, Canada.

Although he has not performed the procedure himself, because he is not a surgeon, Dr. Campbell coauthored a study of SSPE and its treatment in Canada that was recently published in *BMC Pediatrics*. He says the procedure of placing an Ommaya reservoir should not be hard to explain to patients or their parents. The selection of interferon or another drug is somewhat more complicated, mostly because there is little hard evidence about what treatment works best in these cases.

"The medical treatments are largely empirically based or at best [based on] observational studies leaving a great deal of uncertainty about the best management strategy. However, given the disease has a devastating outcome, it would often happen that patients would receive aggressive therapy as did the patients in the report we published. My experience in real clinical medicine over time is that with some patience and thoughtful explanation, real informed consent can be achieved even in the face of the most complex decisions," Dr. Campbell says.

Michael Vassilyadi, M.D., a neurosurgeon at the University of Ottawa and the Children's Hospital of Eastern Ontario in Ottawa, Canada, recalls a procedure similar to the one described on *House, M.D.*

"It was a six-year-old girl with a history of measles," Dr. Vassilyadi remembers. The girl developed myoclonic seizures like those that grabbed the attention of Dr. House. Anticonvulsant medication and oral antiviral drugs did not stabilize the girl's condition, so the medical team decided to try intraventricular interferon treatment.

"I explained the procedure to the patient's father, as well as the risks and complications that included infection, intracranial hemorrhage, and stroke that may create further neurological deterioration," Dr. Vassilyadi says.

"Once the procedure was clearly presented to the father, with illustrations being extremely useful, he understood well and consented. What is required is ample time to provide the explanation in a comfortable environment where everyone is seated, ample time to allow understanding of the procedure and the inherent risks involved, and ample time to respond to the father's questions in a nonrushed fashion."

Dr. Vassilyadi also notes that the surgical procedure to put an Ommaya reservoir in place is relatively straight forward for an average pediatric neurosurgeon.

In addition to painting a frightening and incomplete picture for the patient's parents in "Paternity," Foreman apparently never offered the parents any information about alternatives to the intraventricular interferon therapy he recommended. There are several different drugs that are used to treat SSPE. Even when a physician thinks one choice is superior, a patient needs to know the pros and cons of the various options in order to be able to make a truly informed decision.

Although it seems most physicians would be able to explain this SSPE treatment strategy to patients, the scene illustrates broader shortcomings of current informed consent practices. Many patients, particularly those with weak literacy skills or who speak English as a second language, have trouble adequately understanding even routine medical information and concepts.

An article in an American Cancer Society journal cited a study that reported patients with low literacy skills often do not understand basic terms like screening, colon, tumor . . . or even cure.

The Centers for Disease Control and Prevention, along with other health institutions, recommends that consent forms should aim for a sixth-grade reading level. But achieving that standard, while not oversimplifying the information, presents a difficult challenge.

A survey published in the *New England Journal of Medicine* found that consent forms are usually harder to understand than they are supposed to be. Michael K. Paasche-Orlow, M.D., M.P.H., and his colleagues went to the web sites of over a hundred U.S. medical schools and compared the readability standards listed by the schools with examples of consent-form templates also found on the same medical school web sites. Overall, the actual forms were almost three grade levels more difficult to read than they should have been. That is, if the school standard was that a consent form should be written at a sixth-grade level, the template provided for researchers at the school actually would require patients to have the ability to read at the ninth-grade level.

And when a committee of the American Medical Association published a report on health literacy in the *Journal of the American Medical Association* that, among other recommendations, urged physicians to do a better job of tailoring information to the needs of the patient, some readers quickly pointed out that the journal's own "Patient Page" generally required a twelfth-grade reading level, exceeding the reading ability of the average adult in the United States. The committee members acknowledged the problem. They said they were revising the "Patient Page" to make it easier to read.

Even when physicians do a good job explaining the facts and options so that their patients understand the choices, there is often a tug-of-war between aggressive medical tactics and personal values . . . between doing everything possible to beat the disease and moderating the intensity of the battle, in order to satisfy other concerns or desires of the patient.

That difficult balance comes into sharp focus at the end of life. A review of leading U.S. hospitals by Dartmouth Medical School researchers found wide variations in the amount of medicine deployed during the final six months of patients' lives. In some hospitals, patients averaged less than ten days in the hospital during the final six months of their lives, while in other hospitals the average hospital stay totaled almost a full month.

All the hospitals had top-notch staffs that were presumably equally knowledgeable about the abilities and limitations of medical treatment. And the hospital statistics were adjusted to take into account the age, sex, and illness of the patients.

There was also just as much variation in the place of death. Given a choice, many patients prefer to go home when it becomes apparent that continued intensive hospital treatment is not likely to produce substantial improvements in either health or longevity. But despite having essentially the same medical options available, the choices about continuing aggressive care right up to the end or instead spending the final days with friends and family in familiar surroundings were very different at different hospitals. In some hospitals, five out of six patients go home, while in other hospitals more than half the patients die in the hospital.

Choices about care at the close of life, and when it is time to lay down the arsenal of modern medical technology, rest on the values held by patients and how those values are honored by physicians.

Dr. House, meanwhile, seems to have little concern about the values patients hold, if they conflict with his judgment.

In the first episode, the patient was tired of being bombarded by one draining treatment after another.

"I just want to die with a little dignity," she says.

Dr. House explodes. "There's no such thing! Our bodies break down, sometimes when we're ninety, sometimes before we're even born, but it always happens and there's never any dignity in it. I don't care if you can walk, see, wipe your own ass. It's always ugly, always," he yells at her.

In "Damned If You Do" (1-05), a patient who is also a nun wants to check out of the hospital.

"This illness is a test of my faith," the nun says. "If it's His will to take me, it doesn't matter where I am. I can accept that."

Dr. House doesn't like having his advice rejected, and he goes on the offensive.

"Does anybody believe anything you say? You're not accepting. You're running away. Just like you always do," he retorts.

"First and foremost, Dr. House's attitudes with patients would never ever, ever be tolerated in any organization; and certainly not Princeton. That is just absolutely outrageous," says Joanne Ritter-Teitel, Ph.D., R.N. Dr. Ritter-Teitel is the chief nursing officer at the University Medical Center at Princeton, New Jersey, just around the corner from the fictional location of Dr. House's Princeton-Plainsboro Teaching Hospital.

She says that patients and families would be at her door, and in the offices of other hospital administrators, demanding strong action against any physician who acted the way Dr. House does.

"I don't care what kind of cures the man could perform, in Princeton or in any hospital today, that kind of bedside behavior would never be tolerated. Never. He would be sent to a school for disruptive physicians. He would be sent for all sorts of training to help resolve that behavior; that would not be tolerated," she says.

Dr. House is not only rude and brash; he will even lie in order to get a patient to agree to a test or treatment.

In "Poison" (1-08), Dr. House wants to give a patient an experimental and potentially dangerous treatment. The patient's mother is not convinced. So he has Chase impersonate a CDC scientist in order to prevent the mother of a patient from getting a second opinion that might differ from his own.

In "Detox" (1-11), Dr. House has a complicated rationale for recommending a risky treatment. But rather than respect the ability of the patient's father to understand his reasoning, Dr. House orders Cameron to lie to the father, so he will comply and give consent.

While lying to patients is a clear violation of ethical principles, leaving patients out of the loop is unfortunately common. In 1999, Clarence H. Braddock III, M.D., M.P.H., and his colleagues published an analysis in the *Journal of the American Medical Association* that reported few physicians appear to involve their patients in clinical decision-making. The researchers taped over a thousand doctor-patient encounters involving dozens of physicians and surgeons. According to the researchers' standards, less than one decision in ten completely involved the patient. And among over 200 encounters that dealt with complex decisions, only one decision completely involved the patient.

To Dr. House, the right choice is always clear and beyond debate. He believes he knows better than his patients what is in their best interests. And so despite his medical oath, Dr. House apparently feels justified doing whatever it takes to get patients to bend to his will.

## Mother or Fetus?

Weighing the risks and benefits of cancer treatment is difficult enough for any patient, but when the patient is a pregnant woman, the complexity and trauma of making choices multiplies.

In "Baby and Bathwater" (1-18), a young woman with neurological and other symptoms learns that she is experiencing a paraneoplastic syndrome caused by small-cell lung cancer. She is not a smoker. She is also twenty-eight weeks pregnant. Wilson advises the parents to have the child delivered by Caesarean section immediately, so the mother can begin treatment with chemotherapy and radiation.

Although such cases are rare, they do occur.

John C. Ruckdeschel, M.D., the director of the Barbara Ann Karmanos Cancer Institute in Detroit, Michigan, says paraneoplastic syndromes are the first sign of lung cancer in about 5 percent of the cases he sees.

"They are very confusing syndromes. I've had patients as young as their late twenties, who were nonsmokers," Dr. Ruckdeschel says. "It's something that does happen and it's something that physicians have a bad tendency to miss, because they are not looking for it. People who don't smoke can still get lung cancer, especially women."

He says he usually finds that the patients have been exposed to secondhand smoke at home or at work, although sometimes the cause of a lung cancer is never determined.

On average, Dr. Ruckdeschel says lung cancer patients who have paraneoplastic syndromes as the first symptoms have a poorer prognosis than other lung cancer patients.

He sees pregnant women with cancer a couple of times a year. Indeed, such cases are usually handed off to specialists at major cancer centers because of the complexity, both of the treatment and of the personal choices some patients must make.

Fortunately, in the real world, the patients and spouses rarely have to choose between the life of the mother and the survival of the fetus. In the third trimester, after about twenty-seven weeks, it is usually reasonably safe to begin treatment without risking substantial harm to the fetus.

"The data would suggest that if you are in the third trimester, the chances of causing significant cognitive or developmental problems for the fetus are extremely low. In the first or second trimester, the odds are quite a bit higher," Dr. Ruckdeschel says. "What we would tend to do if we had a cancer that required treatment, and we couldn't put it off for a month or two, we would treat with the baby in utero at this stage and monitor the baby for signs of fetal distress, and we might be able to nurse that kid along, right to a normal-term delivery. I would not feel compelled, with a third trimester baby, to go in and do a C-section delivery at that moment."

He says he and his colleagues have successfully used relatively aggressive chemotherapy during the third trimester. Even radiation therapy can be used on a pregnant woman, if the beam can be focused to limit exposure of the fetus.

Also, waiting a bit, even weeks, is not unreasonable in most cases of cancer during pregnancy. Dr. Ruckdeschel notes that cancer is a long process.

"A week or two is not a problem with respect to the overall biology of the cancer," he says. "Waiting a week is going to be a trivial issue here, if some vital organ is not being pressed on."

Chemotherapy and radiation are extremely hazardous to the fetus early in pregnancy, particularly during the second month, when major organs are beginning to form. Dr. Ruckdeschel says that in every case he has handled, patients in the first trimester have decided to terminate the pregnancy. But it is never an easy decision.

"These are all difficult cases. They require knowing the patient well, sitting down with the patient and saying, 'Here's the situation, the odds that we are not just going to harm the fetus, but kill the fetus, are extremely high'," he says.

"You are taking a relatively young person, who is in one of the happier moments of her life, who is not expecting this, all of a sudden her whole world has fallen apart. But when the survival of the mother becomes an issue and there is no chance for the baby, usually the husband and wife will come to the conclusion that's the right thing to do. They will struggle with it and it may haunt them to a degree, but generally they will opt to save the life of the mother."

If it is possible to delay treatment or it appears that the risks to the fetus are reasonable, then parents usually opt to maintain the pregnancy.

For patients with small-cell lung cancer however, no matter what choice is made, the long term prognosis is poor.

"Even with treatment, the chances of curing that are probably less than two percent. The chance of getting a year or two remission is pretty good, but they are not going to have a normal life," Dr. Ruckdeschel says. "When this is suddenly slapped on you, and you are young, you'll take even a small chance of cure, and that's not unreasonable. I would give them every encouragement to shoot for that."

Other types of cancer also are discovered in women who are pregnant. A recent meeting of international experts reviewed studies of breast cancer during pregnancy. The experts reported that the pregnant patients did as well as patients who were not pregnant. Most cases of breast cancer in pregnant women are treated successfully.

In general, breast cancer surgery can be performed during pregnancy. Several chemotherapy drugs have also been used, though treatment may be delayed until the pregnancy is at least three months along. Radiation is not usually used until after the baby has been delivered. Overall, it does not appear that breast cancer during pregnancy would create any urgent conflicts between the health of the mother and the fetus.

Obstetrician Eytan R. Barnea, M.D., who coedited the textbook *Cancer and Pregnancy*, says that by the time a pregnancy enters the third trimester, the fetus can usually be delivered, if necessary, to avoid conflicts with the mother's cancer treatment.

"Making really hard-core decisions about the survival of the fetus can be made earlier and earlier," he says. "So when the decision is made whether you treat the woman for her cancer or you deliver the fetus first, it comes down to when there is viability versus no viability. And viability can now be accomplished after twenty-seven or twenty-eight weeks."

Dr. Barnea says that risks to the fetus are highest early in the pregnancy. Concerns about toxicity of chemotherapy or radiation are highest during week five to week eight of gestation. If treatment cannot be delayed for at least a few weeks, then termination may be the only option at that early point.

During the second trimester, the fetus has a better chance of withstanding chemotherapy, and even radiation therapy may be possible, if the fetus can be shielded. However, at this stage of pregnancy, delivering the baby is not an option without waiting at least eight to ten weeks.

Dr. Barnea says invasive cervical cancer discovered midway through a pregnancy could present a difficult choice.

"I have not myself had to make this kind of decision, but there are cases in the literature of women with invasive cervical cancer who need an immediate hysterectomy, the pregnancy needs to be terminated, the woman needs to have radiation. If you look at the literature, those are very difficult decisions," he says.

Even in cases of cervical cancer, there are reports of successful treatment that allowed the pregnancy to continue or preserved the woman's ability to become pregnant after treatment. Most cervical cancers discovered during pregnancy are at an early stage. A review of current medical knowledge by Carolyn Muller, M.D., and Harriet Smith, M.D., at the University of New Mexico Health Sciences Center found that, "There is significant evidence that delay in treatment of early stage cancer is not likely to have a deleterious effect on the mother, and that delay of treatment until fetal maturity in a desired pregnancy is a reasonable course of action."

However, they reported that there is little information to guide physicians and patients in making difficult choices in cases of more advanced cancer.

Fortunately, advanced cervical cancer is already rare in the United States and other developed nations thanks to Pap smear screening. And the number of cases around the world may drop dramatically in coming decades, because of a new vaccine against the types of sexually transmitted human papillomaviruses that are the leading cause of cervical cancer.

---

It should be noted that Dr. House is just as willing to lie to his colleagues as he is to his patients. In "Control" (1-14), he misled an organ transplant committee, in order to get his patient to the top of the waiting list. He did not tell the committee members that the patient's heart had been damaged because she abused ipecac as part of an eating disorder. The information might have hurt his patient's chances to get a new heart in time.

As it turned out, because of his deceit, his patient was put ahead of others who were also waiting for new hearts. Because there aren't enough donated organs for all the people who need them, many patients die each year waiting for the pager beep or cell phone call that never comes.

So although Dr. House's patient did receive a new heart and a chance at longer life, someone else on the waiting list did not.

Dr. House also fudged the facts about a patient in order to have her considered for an experimental cancer treatment in "Babies and Bathwater" (1-18). And in "The Socratic Method" (1-06), he injected alcohol into his patient's liver tumor, dehydrating it and causing it to shrink temporarily. The stunt fooled a surgeon into believing the tumor was smaller and easier to remove than it actually was. Dr. House got what he wanted, even if truth was an incidental casualty.

Sometimes, Dr. House violates the law. When he learned that his fifteen-year-old patient in "Skin Deep" (2-13) had had sex with her father, he decided not to immediately report it. In New Jersey, anyone who has reason to believe that child abuse has occurred must report it. The maximum penalty for failing to make a report is six months in jail.

While the laws vary from state to state, physicians and other health care workers are typically included in the language of mandatory reporting requirements. Those requirements mean that when a physician suspects child abuse, he or she has a legal duty to file a report; there is no allowance for personal preferences.

Dr. House offered the excuse that the father was also his patient and so anything the father told him was privileged and could not be revealed to the authorities. Even if the father had been his patient (a questionable claim), doctor-patient confidentiality does not prevent reporting child abuse.

In the episode, Cameron told Cuddy about the incest allegation. Cuddy followed the law and notified the authorities. But the result was not what Cameron expected.

A state worker came right over and spoke to the father and then to the daughter. She passed Cameron on the way out.

"That was quick. What's gonna happen?" Cameron asked.

"What did you think was going to happen?" the state worker replied.

"The father had sex," Cameron started to reply.

"Do you have any medical evidence of that?"

"He admitted it."

"He denies the conversation ever took place. She denies it, too. I'm sure you meant well." The state worker turns and walks away, seeming to dismiss the allegations as a waste of her time.

An allegation that a father had sex with his fifteen-year-old daughter would not be tossed aside so casually, according to Andy Williams, a spokesman for the New Jersey Department of Human Services. While it indeed may be difficult to prove abuse when both parties deny it happened, he says investigators would typically interview anyone else who might have information. That means Dr. House would be interviewed, along with other family members, friends, teachers, and so on. Although Dr. House may not have followed the mandatory reporting law, Williams says he does not recall hearing of a case in which a physician was actually prosecuted for a failure to report child abuse.

Oh, and when the state worker asked Cameron for medical evidence, Cameron could have said that an examination would show the girl was sexually active, thus providing some support for the abuse allegations, while undercutting the child's denial.

A fifteen-year-old girl is too young to consent to sex; it's considered statutory rape. If family services staff suspect a crime may have occurred, the investigator's report would probably be forwarded to law enforcement officials.

## Conflicts of Interest

One component of putting the welfare of patients first is avoiding conflicts with other influences, including money or prestige. Friction between the ideals of medicine and the pressures of industry is increasingly intense.

Dr. House captured one facet of such conflicts in his battle with Edward Vogler over a speech. In the episode "Role Model" (1-17), Vogler is both the chairman of the board of Princeton-Plainsboro Teaching Hospital and the owner of a pharmaceutical company. He asks Dr. House to give a speech praising a new heart disease drug the company is selling. House resists, in part because he doesn't think the new medicine is much better than similar, less expensive medicines. But when Vogler says he'll have to fire one of his staff if he doesn't give the speech, House relents. Sort of. In the end, Dr. House's sense of honesty and his dislike of being ordered around win out: He mocks the drug and embarrasses Vogler in front of an influential audience.

Pharmaceutical and medical device companies cherish the support of prominent physicians. They pay them to be consultants, to give speeches and write articles, and sometimes these payments rival or even exceed the physicians' regular salaries. The National Institutes of Health has been embroiled in struggle over a revised policy on outside payments. A report in the *Los Angeles Times* in 2003 kicked off the debate about NIH policies when it chronicled a list of top researchers who, in addition to their government salaries, were collecting payments from outside sources that over a period of several years totaled hundreds of thousands of dollars each.

When a more restrictive policy was first announced, some leading researchers and others complained, saying that if the limits on outside income were too strict, talented scientists would abandon public agencies and go to work for private industry. The final revised rules ban outside consulting for industry and restrict how much stock in medical industry companies top NIH staffers can hold.

Leading medical journals also are scrutinizing the influence of industry funding and other conflicts. Journal editors are concerned that research articles submitted to them might not always be what they appear; just as Dr. House's speech was not originally going to be what he really thought, but what someone with financial influence over him wanted him to say.

As the editors of the *Journal of the American Medical Association* wrote in an editorial in 2005: "The need for transparency in reporting the financial conflicts of interest of authors and the relationships between investigators and funding sources has never been greater and is essential to help maintain confidence and trust in the scientific integrity of medical research articles."

Any author who wants a paper considered for publication in the journal must provide the following information:

> **Financial Disclosure.** Please check the appropriate box(es) below (applies to the past five years and foreseeable future):
>
> ☐ I have no relevant financial interests in this manuscript.
>
> ☐ I certify that all financial and material support for this research and work are clearly identified in the manuscript.
>
> ☐ I certify that all my affiliations with or financial involvement (e.g., employment, consultancies, honoraria, stock ownership or options, expert testimony, grants or patents received or pending, royalties) with any organization or entity with a financial interest in or financial conflict with the subject matter or materials discussed in the manuscript are disclosed completely here.[1]

Other leading medical journals now have similar disclosure requirements. They do not prohibit research funding from commercial interests, but they want it all out in the open.

1. Authorship Responsibility, Financial Disclosure, Copyright Transfer, and Acknowledgment, *Journal of the American Medical Association* 295 (1) (January 4, 2006):111.

Dr. House expressed concern about commercial influence affecting the care of patients as soon as he first heard that Vogler, the wealthy head of a pharmaceutical company, had become chairman of the board of Princeton-Plainsboro Teaching Hospital. Specifically, he worried about pressure to recruit patients for clinical trials that would benefit Vogler's company. In "Control" (1-14), Dr. House told Dr. Cuddy that Vogler's influence would make the hospital begin acting more like a pharmaceutical company. He worried that doctors would begin pressuring patients into making the wrong choices.

In addition to worrying about marketing spin creeping into medical research reports, the journals are also concerned about industry sponsors trying to bury, sometimes literally, bad news about new products. The *New England Journal of Medicine* chastised researchers involved in a study of the Vioxx pain reliever after it was revealed that the deaths of some patients were not included in a research article that the journal published. Vioxx was pulled off the market by its manufacturer, Merck, after reports of an unexpected number of heart attack deaths among users began to pile up.

The medical journal editors were angered the generally positive research article submitted to them did not include all of the patient death data. The authors said those deaths occurred after a predetermined cut-off date. But the journal editors maintained that the lack of this information misled them and readers.

Another way to potentially skew information about a new drug or device is to do multiple research studies, but then release only the results of the trials that produced favorable results. Although private companies have to follow laws regulating human experimentation, there has not been any requirement that trial results be made public.

In 2004 a group representing leading medical journals, called the International Committee of Medical Journal Editors, announced a new policy. Clinical trials would have to be publicly registered in advance, if the researchers wanted their results to be considered for publication. That way companies could not wait to see the results before deciding whether or not to reveal that a study was being done. The clinical trial registry requirement is intended to be one more tool to fight the selective reporting of information that is favorable to a company's products.

It's a fact that speeches by leading physicians, like the one Vogler pressured Dr. House to make, and studies published in medical journals are vital to the marketing campaigns of drug and device manufacturers. These marketing campaigns are well financed and expertly managed.

In "Sports Medicine" (1-12), Foreman has a fling with a pharmaceutical saleswoman. She also treats the rest of the gang to a nice dinner, while slipping in references to her company's products.

"If the patient decides to go the dialysis route, we've got some product you should check out," she says. Then she goes on to invite them to a medical conference in Bermuda, where the program is heavy on sun and scuba, with only a short lecture to make it a "work" trip.

Dr. House suddenly appears, makes an excuse to get rid of the saleswoman for a moment, and then tells the team that she is just using them in order to get to him, because he has the power to influence which drugs are used in the hospital.

In 2002 the Pharmaceutical Research and Manufacturers of America (PhRMA) adopted a voluntary marketing code for its members that limits, but does not prohibit gifts to doctors. However, it says that gifts should be something that benefits patients; so something useful in a clinic, such as a calendar or a model of an organ would be okay, but a round of golf would not be. Trips and some entertainment are condoned, if it is in connection with consulting work or training for speakers or consultants. The code continues to allow sales representatives to buy meals for physicians, like the one depicted on *House, M.D.*

According to the pharmaceutical industry, more than $25 billion is spent annually to promote medicines. Most of that, about $16 billion, is the value of "free" samples given to physicians. About $6 billion a year is aimed directly at physicians. Despite the voluntary marketing code, a recent article in the *Journal of the American Medical Association* raised questions about industry marketing practices and outlined how some of those billions are spent:

"The following list, while not exhaustive, indicates the interactions with industry that must be addressed: gifts, even of relatively small items, including meals; payment for attendance at lectures and conferences, including online activities; CME (Continuing Medical Education) for which physicians pay no fee; payment for time while attending meetings; payment for travel to meetings or scholarships to attend meetings; payment for participation in speakers bureaus; the provision of ghostwriting services; provision of pharmaceutical samples; grants for research projects; and payment for consulting relationships."

The authors argued that all gifts to physicians, no matter how small, should be prohibited. And they recommended that the "free sample" system be replaced by vouchers given directly to low-income patients, in order to take physicians out of the promotional effort.

The American Medical Student Association also urges those studying to be doctors to resist the goodies offered by industry sales representatives, even pens with logos or sandwiches. The association's PharmFree project is meant to reduce industry involvement in the daily life of physicians.

## Bad Attitude

Why does Dr. House follow his own course and dismiss the standards of others? Is it just because he knows, or at least believes, that he is smarter than everyone else? Does being right about the diagnosis justify blasting through various ethical and legal standards in pursuit of a cure? Is it his own moral compass that leads him to sabotage the marketing moves of drug salespeople and even his own temporary boss, Edward Vogler?

Or is part of his rebelliousness fueled by the gnawing pain of his crippled thigh muscle?

Dr. House explained in the first episode that he suffered an infarction. The patient he was talking to thought he meant he had had a heart attack.

Myocardial infarction is the technical term for a heart attack. Myocardial refers to the muscle of the heart. An infarct is an area of tissue that has died for lack of oxygen. In a typical myocardial infarction, one of the small arteries that supplies blood to the heart muscle is blocked by a clot, often where a cholesterol-laden plaque had built up inside the blood vessel. These blood vessels are not the big ones that the heart pumps blood through to the lungs and the rest of the body. Treatments are aimed at restoring blood flow either by breaking open the clot or bypassing the blockage by grafting a new blood vessel onto the heart.

MIs, as cardiologists often call them, are exceedingly common. Each year in the United States more than a million people a year are hit by a myocardial infarction. But like almost every case depicted on *House, M.D.*, infarctions of skeletal muscles, such as the thigh, are exceedingly uncommon.

Dr. House provided a bit more detail about his thigh damage in "Three Stories" (1-21). He explained that an MRI revealed an aneurysm, which is an abnormal bulge in a blood vessel. Blood in the aneurysm had clotted, cutting off blood flow to his thigh, leading to painful muscle death.

It took three days for physicians to diagnose his thigh infarct. Not that surprising, considering that such skeletal muscle infarcts are not only very rare, but almost all the cases noted in the medical literature involve patients with diabetes or sickle-cell anemia. Dr. House does not seem to have either of those chronic conditions.

Whatever mystery surrounds the cause of his leg injury, Dr. House leaves no doubts about the level of pain it produces. Perhaps the steady consumption of Vicodin he uses to fight the pain also affects his judgment.

The effect of Vicodin and other powerful pain medications on his attitude and his performance is a recurring theme of *House, M.D.* Is he using the drug appropriately or is he addicted? Unfortunately, physician impairment due to the abuse of legal and illegal substances, including alcohol, street drugs, or prescription medicines, is a serious concern.

## Pain, Drugs, and Impaired Physicians

Vicodin is one brand name for a combination pill of hydrocodone and acetaminophen. Hydrocodone is an opioid drug, sharing similarities with morphine. It acts on the opioid receptors in the brain, with pain relief being one of the effects. Acetaminophen is the generic name of the pain reliever in Tylenol.

Brand names for a combination of hydrocodone and acetaminophen:

| | |
|---|---|
| Vicodin | Lortab |
| Anexsia | Norco |
| Co-Gesic | Panacet |
| Lorcet-HD | Zydone |

There's no question that chronic severe pain of the type that afflicts Dr. House is real and that long-term use of pain relievers can help people with such pain function more normally.

Seddon R. Savage, M.S., M.D., the director of the Dartmouth

Center on Addiction, Recovery and Education in Hanover, New Hampshire, says many people with chronic pain function well despite taking powerful pain relievers, including opioids, for long periods. In fact, when the medication is used properly, these patients actually function better than they would without the drugs. Even though these medicines are chemically similar to heroin and opium, there is at least one study that indicates people with pain do not get a "high" with the drugs the way an abuser would. She says that study matches the clinical experience of many pain experts.

A key point in understanding the use of powerful pain relievers is that the dose, by itself, is not the most important fact.

"Dose requirements don't tell you anything about whether somebody has an addiction to medication or is using them therapeutically. There are some people who require only low doses of a medication to get a therapeutic response and there are people who require very high doses of medication to get a satisfactory response," Dr. Savage says.

The important thing to keep an eye on, she says, is how patients function. Are they alert? Are their moods normal? Can they stick to the prescription schedule or do they keep escalating the doses?

In the case of a person who needs strong pain relief indefinitely, like Dr. House, Dr. Savage says she might look to alternatives to Vicodin, because that drug needs to be taken every few hours.

"If somebody has pain twenty-four hours a day and is having to take Vicodin every three hours all day long, they are going to be having variable blood levels. Their blood levels will be going up and down, particularly if they are taking it as they think they need it, rather than on a schedule," she says. "Taking a longer-acting medication once or twice a day that gives them very stable blood levels will provide them that pain relief without periods of withdrawal; they are less likely to have periods where they feel a little fuzzy or cognitively impaired."

There are a variety of sustained-release formulations of morphine and other pain relievers. There are skin patches that release their medicine slowly and steadily throughout the day. There are also drug pumps, some small enough to be placed under the skin, that automatically drip medicine into the patient's body.

In general, pain experts say undertreatment of severe pain is as important, and perhaps more common, a problem as overuse or addiction to pain medications. A key lesson from pain research is to keep fear of addiction in the proper perspective.

"There is healthy fear and there is unnecessary fear," Dr. Savage says. "We see both things at the same time in medical culture today. We have some physicians who really don't have a fear of using opioids and they perhaps have taken to heart a message that opioids don't cause addiction when people have pain. They will prescribe them without always monitoring patients and sometimes get into trouble because of that. And then on the other hand we have physicians who just won't use opioids because they are overly concerned that everyone's going to be turned into an addict.

"Somehow we haven't really found the right balance. I still see that wide divergence of opinion. What we need is a healthy recognition that about ten percent of the population has a lifetime occurrence of addictive disorders, and so about one in ten of the people we treat may have a higher risk than others of developing an addiction."

Like all medicines, powerful pain relievers, such as Vicodin, have risks and benefits. Patients and physicians need to respect the power of the drugs and monitor their use, in order to maximize the benefits while limiting the risks, including addiction.

In 2001 the American Medical Association, the American Pain Society, and more than a dozen other health groups, along with the Drug Enforcement Administration, released *Promoting Pain Relief and Preventing Abuse of Pain Medications: A Critical Balancing Act.* In part, the statement said:

Drug abuse is a serious problem. Those who legally manufacture, distribute, prescribe, and dispense controlled substances must be mindful of and have respect for their inherent abuse potential. Focusing only on the abuse potential of a drug, however, could erroneously lead to the conclusion that these medications should be avoided when medically indicated—generating a sense of fear rather than respect for their legitimate properties. Helping doctors, nurses, pharmacists, other healthcare professionals, law enforcement personnel and the general public become more aware of both the use and abuse of pain medications will enable all of us to make proper and wise decisions regarding the treatment of pain.

The line between appropriate and inappropriate use of pain relievers and other medications or alcohol and other drugs is one that too many physicians cross each year. That fact should not be surprising. After all, physicians are human. Studies of physicians indicate that they get into trouble with substance abuse at about the same rate as people in other professions; that is, a lifetime risk of about one in ten. With almost 600,000 physicians currently practicing in the United States, perhaps as many as 60,000 or so may have some sort of substance abuse problem during their lifetimes.

Even though physicians may not be any more likely than other people to become impaired due to substance abuse, the consequences are far-reaching.

"Physicians like Dr. House, with narcissistic traits, with an attitude that the rules are for everyone but him, are rampant among medical staffs. When you throw drugs on top of that narcissistic, antisocial, curmudgeon, superstar status, you've got yourself a wildfire," says Anderson Spickard, Jr., M.D.

Dr. Spickard is the medical director of the Center for Professional Health in Nashville, Tennessee, and a professor of Medicine and Psychiatry at Vanderbilt University Medical Center. He is the coauthor of the book *Dying for a Drink: What You and Your Family Should Know About Alcoholism.*

Despite years of instruction and experience with prescribing drugs, a physician, even one as skilled at diagnosis as Dr. House, may not see that he or she is standing in the middle of that wildfire.

"Even if he is such an expert at everybody else's illness, he is drastically inexpert about his own potential for addiction," Dr. Spickard says.

Every other month, Dr. Spickard helps teach an intensive course for a dozen physicians on how to regain control over prescription drugs. These physicians have generally been suspended from their practices because they inappropriately dispensed drugs to patients or to themselves, or ran into problems with alcohol. Most of those with personal problems with alcohol and other drugs have already completed rehabilitation treatment.

The physicians who go through the course at the Center for Professional Health have been carefully evaluated and treated, if necessary. But before they can go back to their practices, there are some important lessons to learn, in order to reduce the chances of a relapse: "Have their own physicians; that's number one. It's amazing how few physicians have their own physician. Number two, if they have a narcotic problem themselves, have a physician who knows addiction. Not many physicians are well trained in addictionology. It's a specialty. Number three, avoid mood-altering drugs of all types, because other drugs in the brain seem to trigger the craving for the excess amount of pain medication. Four, go to Narcotics Anonymous meetings and employ the Twelve Steps of NA," Dr. Spickard says.

Although Dr. Spickard and his colleagues have helped hundreds of physicians return to practice over the last several years, there are many more physicians like them still out there.

"We know that about seven percent of a graduating class of

physicians will have an addiction" at some point in their careers, Dr. Spickard says.

"We want to get these guys straightened out. Each one is taking care of fifteen hundred to three thousand patients. Some of them are operating, which is even more scary. Or putting a catheter into your carotid artery or your heart. This is serious business."

Physicians have access to drugs and the legal authority to prescribe them. Where many physicians run into trouble is by trying to treat themselves.

In a medical journal article that he coauthored, Dr. Spickard wrote about one such case.

"A forty-year-old surgeon developed severe flank pain consistent with a renal stone. His friend, an internist, went to his home and gave him an injection of meperidine with instant relief of the pain. The internist friend left a vial of 10 mL of meperidine (100 mg/mL) with his patient with instructions to give himself a shot if the pain returned. The pain returned, and the patient physician gave himself an injection every four hours with immediate relief. His relief was so remarkable and pleasurable that he remembered this feeling even after the renal stone pain subsided. The physician ordered some meperidine for his medical bag and began to medicate himself for even the most trivial discomfort. Soon he was dependent on the medication and began to remove meperidine from his office supplies. Finally, he was confronted by his colleagues and the Impaired Physicians' Committee and was sent to rehabilitation."

A significant point of this story is that the physician was confronted and reported. In an article on impaired physicians, Dr. Spickard notes a statement made by the American Medical Association's Council on Mental Health that "it is the physician's ethical responsibility to take cognizance of a colleague's inability to practice medicine adequately by reason of physical or mental illness including alcoholism and drug dependence."

In the episode "Detox" (1-11), Dr. Cuddy confronted Dr. House about his increasing use of Vicodin. But rather than reporting him or referring him for evaluation, she bet him that he could not quit his pain medication for a week.

Dr. Spickard says he would never recommend challenging a physician to go "cold turkey" as a way to either prove or disprove suspicions of addiction.

"No, because withdrawal symptoms, which are tearing, diarrhea, and all that, can happen with a smaller dose and would not be evidence necessarily of addiction. Withdrawal is not lethal; it's just bothersome with those symptoms. It doesn't prove one way or the other whether the person is addicted," he says.

The pain would probably be severe. Not only would the original pain that led to treatment return, it could be magnified by the withdrawal, leaving the patient in worse shape than before treatment.

While Vicodin withdrawal is not life threatening, suddenly stopping treatment with some drugs, such as short-acting benzodiazepines, can cause serious reactions, including seizures.

If addiction cannot be determined by the dose of drug that is being consumed, where is the line? When the drug seems to become more important than friends, family, job, or other facets of life, that may be addiction.

"Taking more than they should for the condition and suffering consequences from the use or addiction and continuing to do it anyway. Addiction is defined as continuing the use of the medication, or alcohol, despite adverse consequences," Dr. Spickard says.

The warning signs include missing appointments, mistakes in medical orders, frequent or inappropriate anger, and family problems including divorce. Dr. Spickard also notes that physicians who may be addicted may seek a "geographic cure"; that is, moving to another institution, maybe in another city. These physicians may say, and believe, that their problems are due to their supervisors or hospital rules and regulations, rather than their own loss of control over medicines or alcohol and other drugs.

The problem of impaired physicians has been given a great deal of attention within the profession in recent decades. Hospitals are better than they used to be at recognizing and responding to potential problems, although many physicians with possible substance abuse issues still slip by.

The responsiveness of hospital administrations is motivated by more than their sense of obligation to patients and to their colleagues. Health care institutions that fail to take action may be subject to penalties.

"Any hospital administrator would be well aware of the federal regulations about drug use by physicians, and they'd put themselves at great risk by knowing this guy was around and not having him properly assessed by the Physicians Wellness Committee and the Physicians Wellness Program of the institution," Dr. Spickard points out.

The hospital administrator who is supposed to be supervising Dr. House is Dr. Lisa Cuddy, even though she often seems to be just hanging on tight during the wild ride, rather than running the operation. Next we'll look at how hospitals like the fictional Princeton-Plainsboro Teaching Hospital operate.

# Identification of the Impaired Physician

## HIGH RISK CONDITIONS FOR ADDICTION

- Family history of addiction in first-degree relatives
- Access to mood-altering medication, particularly opioids, particularly in anesthesiology
- Domestic breakdown
- Unusual stresses at work

## BEHAVIORS OF ADDICTION

- Use of large quantities of alcohol; frequent drunkenness
- Frequent medical complaints without specific medical diagnosis evident (fatigue, insomnia, indigestion, depression)
- Self-prescribing of sedative-hypnotic, opioid injections
- Neglect of responsibilities (missing appointments, late to rounds)
- Frequent outbursts of anger
- Staff concerns about a colleague's behavior
- Sexual promiscuity
- Driving under the influence citations

## SIGNS OF ADDICTION

- Smell of alcohol on breath
- Ataxic gait
- Slurred speech
- Unexplained tremor
- Disheveled appearance
- Somnolence
- Unexplained weight changes
- Depressed mood

*From P. G. O'Connor and A. Spickard, Jr., "Physician Impairment by Substance Abuse," The Medical Clinics of North America 81(4)(July 1997): 1037–52. Review.*

# EIGHT

# No Doctor Is an Island

As Edward Vogler began his brief tenure as the chairman of the board of Princeton-Plainsboro Teaching Hospital, he had a question for Dr. Cuddy.

"What is a Department of Diagnostic Medicine?"

"That's Dr. House's department," Dr. Cuddy replied. "They deal with cases that other doctors can't figure out."

Vogler is perplexed by Dr. House's idiosyncrasies and challenged by his resistance to Vogler's efforts to run the hospital like any other business.

But even when you look past Dr. House's peculiarities, hospitals are not like any other businesses. The authors of a textbook titled *Health Care USA: Understanding Its Organization and Delivery* highlighted the daunting complexity of modern hospitals. Hundreds or even thousands of people, many of whom have advanced degrees and extraordinary expertise, work together in a highly regulated organization providing customized services to people whose lives are at stake.

"[W]ith so many different kinds of employees and so many inter-related systems and functions, it is a small wonder that they work at all," authors Harry Sultz and Kristina Young wrote.

Hospitals were not always this way. When the United States was established, Sultz and Young point out, hospitals were little more than pesthouses. In the eighteenth century, people did not go to a hospital to be cured; people infected with contagious diseases were sent to hospitals in order to protect the rest of the community. People who had the money to hire physicians usually received treatment at home.

As medical knowledge and practice has changed, and as society has altered its expectations of health care, hospitals have gone through several transformations. It is really only within the last century or so that people began to see hospitals as institutions that provided valuable health care services. Modern health care insurance got its start in the 1930s with prepayment plans that guaranteed a certain number of days of hospital care. After World War II, the nation went on a hospital-building boom. Then as hospital care became increasingly sophisticated and expensive in recent decades, smaller hospitals closed and care of very sick patients became increasingly concentrated in large institutions that could afford the costly tools that physicians like Dr. House employ with such fervor.

There are two principal ways to categorize hospitals: one, by the types of health care services they provide, and two, by their ownership structure. There are three basic types of hospital ownership:

- Not for profit; for example, hospitals owned by religious groups or foundations

- For profit; these hospitals may be part of a chain or independent, but they are meant to make money for their owners

- Public hospitals; these hospitals may be owned and operated by a city or county, or a federal agency, such as the military or the Department of Veterans Affairs.

The types of services and how hospitals go about providing them is not as simple to categorize. In fact, hospitals can be looked at as structures that are built out of an array of programs. For instance, a hospital may have an emergency room, it may have a heart transplant program, and it may provide psychiatric services. But another hospital nearby may have none of these particular services and still be a hospital. Some hospitals are affiliated with medical schools and others are not.

## Princeton-Plainsboro Teaching Hospital

So where does Princeton-Plainsboro Teaching Hospital fit in this hospital spectrum? It does not appear to be a public hospital. After all, Dr. Cuddy hasn't been hauled before a county commission yet. Likewise, there are no symbols of a religious order around the building, so it does not seem to be part of one of the nation's church-affiliated health care systems.

Whether the ownership is a for-profit corporation or a not-for-profit foundation, Princeton-Plainsboro Teaching Hospital seems to stand on its own, without any references to a distant hospital chain headquarters. As the name implies, the hospital is also a training ground for new physicians. However, Dr. House seems to have only occasional contact with students . . . and he treats them with the same disdain he has for his clinic duties.

Indeed, in the first season medical students figured prominently in only two episodes. In "Three Stories" (1-21), Dr. House lectures an auditorium class, but Dr. Cuddy has to bribe him with time off from clinic duty in order to fill in for an ill professor. And then, as if to emphasize his disdain for teaching, Dr. House jumps back and forth between the stories of three patients with severe leg pain. He even goes as far as changing key details as he goes along, seemingly in order to torment the students.

In "Histories" (1-10), a pair of medical students appears in one of the minor side stories. Dr. House is typically gruff, sending them off to get a medical history from a patient without any detailed instructions. Then when the students are confused because the patient tells them each different stories, Dr. House taunts them, seemingly exasperated by their inability to recognize the rare condition that has affected the patient's memory.

Although Princeton-Plainsboro is billed as a teaching hospital, Dr. House seems to view students the way a sports car driver looks at speed bumps.

---

## When Is a Hospital Not a Hospital?

What hospital building stands in for the fictional Princeton-Plainsboro Teaching Hospital in the aerial views sprinkled throughout *House, M.D.*? Well, none really. The building pictured on the series is actually Princeton University's Frist Campus Center. It is named after the family of U.S. Senate Majority Leader Bill Frist (R-TN). Sen. Frist, who is also a physician, is a Princeton alumnus.

Older alumni of Princeton who have not visited the campus recently might not recognize the building at first. The angle usually shown on *House, M.D.* emphasizes a modern expansion that was grafted onto the old Palmer Physical Laboratory building, which was built almost a century ago.

---

Then there is Dr. House's relationship with the hospital administration, which exaggerates and skews some aspects of how physicians and hospital administrators deal with each other, while capturing the essence of some age-old conflicts. Here again, hospitals are not like other businesses. The CEO of a hospital often does not have total control over the physicians who work there. Certainly, Dr. Lisa Cuddy does not have Dr. House under her control.

Edward Vogler does not understand the relationship. When he took over as chairman of the board of the hospital, he sharply criticized Dr. Cuddy for what he saw as her failure to supervise Dr. House effectively. In the episode "Heavy" (1-16), he tries to demonstrate his power by ordering Dr. House to fire one of his fellows. Dr. House offers to instead reduce all their salaries to save an equivalent amount of money, but Vogler refuses.

Dr. Cuddy doesn't get it, because she thinks Vogler's point is to save money. Dr. House grasps Vogler's true intent . . . to demonstrate his power. Vogler confirms Dr. House's realization, saying that he needs to know that Dr. House will do whatever Vogler asks, no matter how distasteful, and that he wants Dr. House to understand his subservient role. Of course, Dr. House is determined to maintain his star billing in the hospital.

Bruce Traub, C.P.A., has a special perspective on the management dynamics portrayed on *House, M.D.* He is the chief financial officer of the University Medical Center at Princeton, New Jersey. His teaching hospital is just down the road from the fictional location of Princeton-Plainsboro Teaching Hospital, and in many ways could be considered a sort of model for Dr. House's hospital.

"Like most organizations, we have a president and CEO. But parallel to that, you have the elected officers of the medical and dental staff," Traub points out. The officers are elected by the physicians and dentists, not the administration.

"So that's one part of the medical and dental staff leadership. And then within the departments of the hospital you have appointed chairs. For example, you have an appointed chair of the Department of Medicine, the Department of Surgery, Psychiatry, and so forth."

This parallel hierarchy of the medical staff is one of the features that make hospitals different from other businesses. The department chairs and the medical/dental officers meet at least monthly with the leaders of the hospital administration. And while they may routinely work together to manage any issues that come up, including physician behavior, the division of responsibilities and authority means that hospital administrators cannot simply issue orders or make unilateral decisions about things that affect physicians. Vogler's insistence that physicians obediently carry out his instructions is something about which most hospital CEOs can only secretly dream.

What's more, at most hospitals in the real world, even though physicians work in the building and use the hospital's facilities and other resources, they are usually not employees the way clerks or maintenance workers are. And yet, since doctors decide who is admitted to the hospital, they are responsible for bringing in business. Traub says that in some ways the physicians are the hospital's sales force.

"So we have limited control over our 'sales force'; what they do, how they refer patients to us," Traub says. "We spend all the money to provide the resources for them to do their jobs here, yet they actually make their money from their own billings to patients, not from a paycheck from us. So it's a unique relationship that I don't think has a parallel in any other industry."

That fact does not mean physicians are free to do whatever they want. In order to maintain their privileges to practice at the hospital, physicians must adhere to bylaws and procedures that address major issues, such as patient safety, and also smaller matters, such as when doctors should wear white lab coats.

## Of White Coats and "Functionless" Ties

When new chairman of the board of Princeton-Plainsboro Edward Vogler catches his first glimpse of Dr. House in "Control" (1-14), he notices something amiss. Dr. House is not wearing a white lab coat. Dr. Cuddy shrugs off Dr. House's aversion to the standard white coat, but Vogler seems unconvinced that exceptions should be made to the dress code.

The white lab coat is as much a symbol of medicine as the stethoscope. But dress codes requiring physicians to wear lab coats are not as universal as they once were. In a commentary in the *Archives of Internal Medicine*, gastroenterologist Lawrence J. Brandt, M.D., mused about the increasingly casual attire of young physicians and medical students.

Dr. Brandt wrote that as he looked out over the audience for an annual lecture he gives to medical students at the Albert Einstein College of Medicine in the Bronx, New York, he saw a stark contrast to the starched white-coated clean-cut student body he was part of in an earlier decade.

"Obviously, these men and women were not aware of or chose to ignore Hippocrates' advice that the physician should 'be clean in person, well dressed, and anointed with sweet-smelling unguents,'" Dr. Brandt wrote.

He then undertook a review of the medical literature, not for the usual research findings on gastrointestinal issues, but for articles about medical dress codes and attire. Dr. Brandt found a rich mix of writings that explored both the practical and symbolic dimensions of physician attire. The white coat is a symbol of both sanitation and authority. It speaks to both the patient and to colleagues. And as Dr. Brandt noted, the ample pockets are useful for carrying everything from stethoscopes to textbooks to the latest PDAs full of downloaded medical data.

## No Doctor Is an Island

Not all the symbolism is beneficial. The phenomenon of "white coat hypertension" is well documented. The term refers to the fact that some people have higher blood pressure when they are checked in a doctor's office or clinic than when the readings are taken at home, away from any white-coated physicians. Indeed, there is substantial concern that white coat hypertension may skew the treatment of some patients. In response, when physicians suspect patients may have high blood pressure, they are increasingly sending them home with blood pressure monitors, in order to get an accurate picture of blood pressure throughout a normal day, rather than just a snapshot in the clinic. Of course, white coat hypertension is not triggered merely by the sight of a doctor's coat. It probably involves a psychological response to the general stress some people feel when visiting their doctors' offices.

There is no law or other regulation that requires doctors to wear white coats. Dress codes at some hospitals and other health care institutions may be prominently enforced, while at other hospitals the dress code may be informal or little known.

At the Stanford University Medical Center in California, the dress code of one program says, in part:

> White lab coats will be worn by staff members providing direct patient care, except in areas where other protective clothing is required, such as BMT [the bone marrow transplant area]. In out-patient areas, psych, and the rehab unit, lab coats are not required. Consult with your clinical instructor about clothing in the area you will be assigned.
>
> —Stanford Hospital and Clinics Rehabilitation
> internship program web site

And of course, the rules may vary depending on the status of the wearer. The rules may be stricter for students. The Student Handbook for the Carolinas College of Health Sciences in Charlotte,

North Carolina, states that medical students should wear three-quarter-length white lab coats over street clothes when they are not wearing hospital scrubs or other special clothing.

Dr. Brandt noted in his commentary that surveys of patients tend to show that most, though not all, prefer that their physicians wear white coats. And some surveys indicate patients are more likely to trust a physician wearing a white coat.

In his conclusion, Dr. Brandt wrote:

"It appears that the attire of the health care provider is important to patients across all lines of population and geography studied to date: young or old, child or parent, eastern or western, northern or southern. A neat, clean appearance, however, is more important than attire. Among professional apparel, the name tag and the white coat are most preferred by patients. In general, physicians are more conservative in their opinions about their attire than are their patients. Older patients especially, but individuals in all age ranges, tend to favor more formal dress."

Some studies, however, raise some practical issues. Sometimes the coats are not so sanitized, according to studies that found various microbes lurking on physicians' coats. And neckties are under assault in some corners. The British Medical Association (BMA) created a stir when it classified neckties as "functionless clothing" that may do more harm than good.

A summary of the BMA report stated:

"Certain clothes such as ties are rarely laundered but worn daily, commonly outside the healthcare environment. Ties perform no beneficial function in patient care and have been shown to be colonised by pathogens. They are regularly handled by the owner and come into contact with numerous objects. Ties have the potential, therefore, to act as a vector for the transmission of HCAIs [health care associated infections]."

Bottom line: Lose the ties . . . wash other clothing frequently and, where possible, change clothes when leaving the patient care areas.

Oh, speaking of washing . . . crusaders fighting the spread of infections within hospitals keep hammering away at health care professionals to always, always wash their hands between every patient visit, in order to avoid transferring microbes from one patient to another. They have had varying degrees of success with these campaigns. Often experts recommend patients try to help enforce the standards by watching to see if their doctors or other health care providers wash their hands before touching them. Although it may be difficult to question a physician or nurse, they say: Don't be shy, ask your doctor to wash before touching.

One episode of *House, M.D.* was based on the spread of a lethal virus within the neonatal unit. In "Maternity" (1-04), however, the source of the infection was not a physician or nurse, but a volunteer who unknowingly carried the virus from baby to baby as she delivered stuffed animals.

---

Shrugging off a dress code is one thing, but most hospital administrations would respond quickly if a physician tried to make an end-run around a decision of the hospital transplantation committee, in order to get a new heart for his patient, as Dr. House did in "Sex Kills" (2-14), or used an injection of alcohol to temporarily shrink his patient's liver tumor, in order to fool a surgeon into agreeing to operate on her, as he did in "The Socratic Method" (1-06).

"If it's something of that magnitude, it is heard about that day. Usually it is reported by another physician, maybe directly to the CEO," Bruce Traub says.

The University Medical Center at Princeton recently added a physician to its administrative leadership. As at most hospitals, this vice president of Medical Affairs would be on the front lines of any potential disciplinary action or other serious issue involving a physician.

In "The Mistake" (2-08), Chase went before a "peer review committee" that judged his actions in the case of a patient who died. After hearing his side of the story, the committee ruled that Chase lied to his superiors and the patient's brother. But the committee members took into account the fact that Chase had just been told his father had died. They said this unexpected jolt mitigated his failure to properly follow-up with the patient, and so they left intact his privileges to practice medicine at the hospital.

Then the committee surprised Dr. House by announcing that allegations about his conduct were serious enough to warrant temporary restriction of his privileges. For a month, Foreman was put in charge of Dr. House.

In real hospitals, physicians are reviewed by both their peers and administrators according to the bylaws of the medical staff and other rules.

"Ultimately there is a governance process," Traub says. "If somebody is not acting appropriately, it goes before the Executive Committee of the medical and dental staff. We as administrators can request that something be brought up before that group; or a physician can request that it be brought up before that group."

Several different types of groups may be involved in the scrutiny of a physician's actions. Questions about ethics may be brought before an advisory committee that includes members of the community. A bioethics committee usually doesn't have direct disciplinary authority, but it does have input to the process. There also are performance-improvement committees that can meet on short notice to evaluate other aspects of a physician's practice.

These committees, and even the top medical staff officers and administrators, cannot abruptly fire a physician without due process, but if necessary, they can take quick actions to protect patients.

"There is a series of meetings and hearings that would be held, all the way up to the board. A physician could be suspended, if he or she did something outrageously unsafe to a patient. That could bring a suspension pending an investigation. But it's a fair hearing process in which members of the medical staff and experts within the department would be convened to hear the physician on that particular question," says Joanne Ritter-Teitel, Ph.D., R.N. She is the chief nursing officer of the University Medical Center at Princeton, a position that is part of the hospital's administration.

"It is not an uncommon practice to send a physician for counseling or a course on communication," she says. As discussed earlier, sometimes these referrals to counseling or training are part of the response to concerns about whether a physician is impaired by alcohol or other drugs, including prescription medications such as Dr. House's beloved Vicodin.

## What Is "Outrageously Unsafe"?

How about experimenting on a comatose patient? In "Distractions" (2-12), Dr. House injects drugs into a patient who is in a coma, in order to satisfy his curiosity about the effectiveness of an experimental migraine treatment. He isn't secretive about it, showing no shame when Dr. Cuddy interrupts him. When she realizes that he has induced and then attempted to treat a migraine in a person who is unconscious and completely unable to give consent, she is dumbfounded. She asks Dr. House if he has ever read an ethical guideline; however, she doesn't take any action, despite having witnessed a blatant violation of a patient's rights.

After Dr. Cuddy shrugs off the criminal assault, she then moves on to the issue she first came to see Dr. House about: a memo carrying her signature ... apparently forged by Dr. House. He doesn't deny the forgery and then makes a sexually suggestive joke about the appropriate discipline.

Dr. House again acts outrageously, and in direct violation of standard hospital procedures concerning organ donation, when he intrudes on the husband of a dying patient in "Sex Kills" (2-14). He wants to find out whether the victim of a car crash might be a potential organ donor for his patient. Clearly he knows he's skirting the rules, because he slides up to the husband's side wearing camouflage. Well, for Dr. House it is the ultimate camouflage: a white lab coat.

He begins quizzing the husband about whether his wife had any illnesses before her car crash. The husband says she had a fever of 101 degrees. As Dr. House continues to probe, the husband becomes exasperated and bewildered about the connection between his wife's general health and the treatment for her crash injuries.

Then a woman comes up to the tense pair. She says she is the organ procurement coordinator for southern New Jersey. She begins telling the husband that his wife's organs will be treated with care and dignity. The husband just stares at her in shock.

"Her organs?! Laura died?"

It's the transplant coordinator's turn to look shocked.

"I'm sorry. I thought, um. She was just pronounced dead. I thought he was telling you." She gestures to Dr. House.

The husband turns to Dr. House. "What did you want from me?"

"I'm sorry for your loss, but I need your wife's heart." With his reply, Dr. House again demonstrates that he is concerned about his patients only, not those under the care of other physicians.

Dr. House's stealth approach to the dying patient's husband not only created uncomfortable confusion and heightened the anguish of the husband ... it was an almost-perfect example of how not to confront family members with the decision about authorizing organ donation. As a statement from an organ donation advocacy group put it: "It is obvious that what he is doing is very unusual and improper."

---

## Organ Donation: Best Practices

In 2003, the U.S. Department of Health and Human Services established the "Organ Donation Breakthrough Collaborative," in order to save lives by increasing the rates of organ donation.

A report from the group stated that its goals are to

- increase the average conversion rate of eligible donors from the current average of 43 percent to 75 percent in the nation's largest 200 hospitals;

- increase donations by up to 1,900 donors per year;

- increase transplantations by 6,000 per year; and

- help save lives of thousands of people each year and prevent up to seventeen deaths per day.

One path toward those goals was to study some of the programs around the country that demonstrate the greatest success. The review included an evaluation of how health care staff members approach family members. The group found that the programs assigned the task of raising the subject of organ donation to different people. Some programs leave the job to a full-time representative of the regional organ procurement organization. Other programs give the delicate job to members of the hospital staff. Despite the different views about who should have the lead responsibility, all these successful programs had clearly defined procedures that involved "close, well-understood, and reliable collaboration."

Families need time to think and prepare themselves both for the death of their loved one and the decision about organ donation; so the staff starts its work well before the patient has died by learning about the family dynamics, how family members are feeling and coping with the situation, and what needs they might have.

The process often can't wait until after the potential donor has been declared dead, because there is usually a very brief window of opportunity to get the family's consent and successfully retrieve and transplant the organs. Even when the potential donor has signed a donor card or has a driver's license notation indicating his or her agreement to be a donor, the family still has veto power at the time of death. So the people designated to talk to the family need to establish a relationship early. By starting to build ties before it is even certain that the patient is going to die, the staff members have an opportunity to demonstrate that their first concern is for the life of the patient and also the needs of the family . . . and that organ donation is a matter that comes up after every attempt to save the patient has been tried.

The group studying best practices noted in its report that the system works best when the people who are responsible for asking families about donation "are not solely focused on 'procuring organs' but on supporting families to come to an informed decision that is right for them." That focus on the needs and desires of families is a trait that seems alien to Dr. House.

Programs that succeed more often when they approach families about organ donation typically

- work as a team to determine the right person or person(s) to raise the issue of donation and make the request;

- ask at the right time, not rushing the family, not asking too soon. It is important to address the family's need and establish trust before discussing donation;

- make sure staff who make the request are specifically trained to ask in the right way.

Doing things right can have substantial rewards. The report said that after one Houston hospital created an organ donation center and staff, consent rates jumped from 48 percent to 68 percent and the number of organ donors during comparable time periods rose from fifty-six to seventy-nine. Since the organs from one donor usually go to several recipients, this one hospital was able to save at least dozens more lives by following a carefully planned process.

To put it another way, just jumping in and confronting the husband of a potential donor, the way Dr. House did in "Sex Kills," typically will fail, and thus cost the lives of many patients who need organ transplants.

---

While Dr. Cuddy appears exasperated by Dr. House's serial recklessness, ultimately she shrugs off each incident. It is extremely unlikely a real hospital administrator in her position would simply let Dr. House slide; no matter how much she likes him or respects his medical skill. In the real world, a hospital and its administrators can suffer serious consequences for permitting a physician to stray too far from standard practices. Myriad outside institutions monitor hospitals and some have the authority to levy heavy fines or even shut down a hospital. Doctors are not the only ones with state licenses; hospitals are licensed, too. And without a license, a hospital is out of business.

## Rules and Regulations

In New Jersey, a hospital like the University Medical Center at Princeton, or the fictional Princeton-Plainsboro Teaching Hospital, must answer to its Board of Trustees, the New Jersey Department of Health and Senior Services, as well as other organizations that monitor and pay for health care in hospitals.

The New Jersey Department of Health and Senior Services is the licensing agency for hospitals in the state. Similar agencies serve that purpose in other states.

According to a statement from the department, it conducts dozens of inspections of hospitals and other health care facilities each year. In addition, the department responds to complaints. The evaluations include reviewing buildings, equipment, and personnel. Hospital policies and procedures are checked to make sure they conform to state laws and regulations. The results of facility inspections done by the New Jersey state inspectors can also affect a hospital's eligibility for reimbursement by federal health care programs, including Medicare, the insurance program that covers people sixty-five and older.

Many of the enforcement actions taken by the state against hospitals are listed on the department's web site. Minor paperwork violations, such as failing to file the right reports on time, may bring a fine of a few hundred or even a couple of thousand dollars. Problems that could affect patient care can bring bigger fines. For instance, the department fined one hospital more than $22,000 in a recent case in which the department ruled that the hospital released a patient with tuberculosis without taking proper steps to make sure the patient would not infect other people in the community.

As in other states, a separate state agency, the New Jersey State Board of Medical Examiners handles licenses and legal sanctions against individual physicians, including those who practice in hospitals.

In "Failure to Communicate" (2-10), Dr. House and Stacy have to fly up to Baltimore, Maryland, to answer questions about his bills for treating patients enrolled in Medicaid, the program that helps to pay for care for millions of low-income Americans. Stacy is able to get the questions essentially to disappear by cajoling the Medicaid investigator into agreeing that Dr. House's handling of the cases was appropriate, even if it didn't always conform to the letter of Medicaid reimbursement rules. The almost-instantaneous resolution of a federal inquiry is a pleasant little fantasy. Federal health care regulations and their enforcement could certainly give the tax code a run for its money in terms of bewildering complexity . . . and anyone who has gone through an IRS audit knows that simple, quick, and favorable solutions are rare, indeed.

One odd element in the premise of this episode was that Dr. House would go to Baltimore to answer the questions. Assuming the matter required a personal interview, he should have gone to Trenton, the capital of New Jersey. Although a large share of Medicaid funding is federal, the program is largely administered by states. It is the states that take the lead on Medicaid fraud investigations.

Boards and agencies of the state and federal governments are not the only ones hospital administrators have to answer to. There are also accrediting agencies. These bodies include groups that oversee medical education. Princeton-Plainsboro Teaching Hospital probably would need to meet the standards of the Association of American Medical Colleges in order to participate in the education of medical students. Then separate accreditation would be required from the Accreditation Council for Graduate Medical Education in order to train interns and medical residents, who are M.D.s at the early stages of their careers.

The Joint Commission on Accreditation of Healthcare Organizations plays an important role in monitoring the quality of hospital treatment, even though it is not a governmental agency and has no regulatory authority. Although the Joint Commission (also known as "Jayco" for its initials JCAHO) cannot directly punish hospitals, government agencies often rely on the results of its inspections and other reports. For instance, a hospital with Joint Commission accreditation may not have to also go through separate certification by the Medicare program. If Joint Commission inspectors were reviewing the accreditation of Princeton-Plainsboro Teaching Hospital, Dr. House would probably be a problem. A short list of concerns might include the following:

- using treatments and running tests without the permission of patients

- lying to patients and coworkers

- verbally abusing and sometimes even striking patients and coworkers who don't agree with his recommendations

- possible impairment due to inappropriate use of Vicodin and other pain medications

- disregarding patient privacy by discussing the details of cases in the clinic and other open areas

- violating a patient's "do not resuscitate" instructions

- violating hospital rules governing the care of patients with immune system disorders, potential organ donors, and others

- searching the homes of patients without permission.

"His personal behaviors are clearly inflammatory, irreverent, and at times even illegal." That is the initial reaction of Peter Angood, M.D., to a list of incidents from episodes of *House, M.D.* Dr. Angood is a vice president of the Joint Commission on Accreditation of Healthcare Organizations and chief patient safety officer of the Joint Commission International Center for Patient Safety.

"There is not one of those that is not outside of the boundaries of regular medical staff guidelines for behavior. Anytime a physician is brought onto the staff of a hospital, they go through a review process and have to substantiate their education, their experience, and their practices," he says. "It's clear the guy has some kind of dependency problem. It's clear that he has a total disrespect for authority or the hierarchy. So his personal behaviors are way, way out of the reality of the true world."

Dr. Angood holds the hospital administration responsible, too.

"The other component is that they portray the tolerance by the hospital in allowing him to continue on; and that just would not occur and does not occur," he says. "In my twenty-five years of practice I have seen changes in the level of tolerance toward what we loosely term disruptive or abusive practitioner behavior. There is very little tolerance now. Almost all institutions have pretty tight human resources and medical staff processing, in terms of not only identifying these individuals but also getting them into a counseling process or getting them out of the system entirely."

The Joint Commission sets standards, such as protecting patient privacy. It is then up to hospitals and other health care facilities to devise and follow procedures that keep them in compliance with those standards. Years may pass between on-site visits by Joint Commission inspectors, but that does not necessarily mean Dr. House would be able to escape notice. Every year, the Joint Commission receives almost 15,000 complaints directly from patients and even hospital staff members. When a complaint comes in, the hospital has to respond.

The response to behavior like the kind Dr. House displays can be much more forceful than what is portrayed on the show.

"You would expect that the hospital, through one of its committees or processes, would have vetted those particular instances and said we're either going to sanction this guy or put somebody else on the case or he's going to go through [privacy] training or see the compliance officer or suspend privileges. And you never see any of that occur on the show, as if the hospital administrators, while they agree that's he's done something outrageous or beyond the rules, [just say] 'Well, it's House,'" says Margaret VanAmringe, the Joint Commission's vice president for public policy and government relations.

"Hospitals are expected to review the competencies of medical staff on a periodic basis. So in the real world, he would come up for reprivileging in an annual review. And at that review, hospitals need to use information to make a decision about regranting him privileges. So if there were a lot of complaints about drug abuse or suspicions, he likely would be asked some very pointed questions and potentially be asked to undergo a medical evaluation," she adds.

The Joint Commission very rarely revokes the accreditation of a hospital. Usually the threat of losing accreditation and the subsequent potential loss of revenue from public and private insurance and other programs is enough to motivate administrators to comply with Joint Commission recommendations. In some cases, though, hospitals choose to voluntarily drop their Joint Commission accreditation. They can remain open without it, if they are able to meet the requirements of government licensing agencies and the standards of public and private health care insurance plans.

## Teamwork

The director of the federal Agency for Healthcare Research and Quality, Carolyn Clancy, M.D., recalls the finale of a set of lecture slides often used by her predecessor, John Eisenberg, M.D. It included images of clinical textbooks and other tools that young doctors have long relied on to learn the trade.

"The other slide that went in this set was a picture of the Marlboro Man. Dr. Eisenberg would say that the myth around training doctors has always been that once you get through training, it's you and your patient and you ride off into the sunset together and you can do what you want. And it's a lie, because that's not what medical practice is like now," she remembers Dr. Eisenberg explaining.

Contrary to the strong theme of Dr. House's individual brilliance, modern medicine is a team sport. Dr. House does employ his fellows, Cameron, Foreman, and Chase to do his grunt work, but this team is not like what most hospital physicians work with.

For example, David Gilbert, M.D., director of Medical Education at Providence Portland Medical Center in Portland, Oregon, says the teams of physicians are varied and extended. Dr. Gilbert, who is a specialist in infectious diseases, like Dr. House, says his hospital uses teams including a senior resident, a first-year resident, and a medical student. They take care of whoever comes into the hospital during their shifts. The younger physicians are supervised by more experienced doctors and they consult with a variety of specialists. Depending on the shift, each medical team may be dealing with anywhere from three to twenty patients at a time, never just one at a time.

One key aspect of *House, M.D.* does capture an important trend in medicine: the growing ranks of physicians who specialize in treating patients in the hospital. Dr. House's work is done entirely within the hospital. He does not have an outside practice seeing patients for routine and continuing care. He takes control during the crisis, and then sends the patients back to their regular physicians.

"The old vision of American medicine was that your regular doctor, like Marcus Welby, would be your doctor wherever you went; in the office and in the hospital. That model doesn't work very well anymore, in part because doctors are extraordinarily busy in the office, and in part because, as the threshold for hospitalization has gone up and up, patients who do end up in hospital tend to be incredibly sick, with a lot of things going on, a lot of specialty consultations, different medications, a lot of complexity," says Robert Wachter, M.D. Dr. Wachter is the chief of the Medical Service at UCSF Medical Center in San Francisco,

California. "So the need for focused expertise and the need for around-the-clock presence has created real value in having a doctor who sort of lives in the place. It's what they read about. It's what they focus on."

A decade ago, Dr. Wachter and his colleague, Lee Goldman, M.D., wrote an article about how changes in medical practice were making it impossible to sustain the old ideal of the primary care physician who can keep tabs on all her patients, whether they come to the clinic or are confined in the hospital. In that article in the *New England Journal of Medicine* they coined a new word for a new kind of physician.

"As a result, we anticipate the rapid growth of a new breed of physicians we call 'hospitalists'—specialists in inpatient medicine—who will be responsible for managing the care of hospitalized patients in the same way that primary care physicians are responsible for managing the care of outpatients," Wachter and Goldman wrote in that article.

Although Dr. House is called a "diagnostician," he really is a hospitalist. And as such, he has a lot of company now. Although the term was invented barely a decade ago, there are now some 15,000 hospitalists in the United States. Dr. Wachter was the first elected president of the Society of Hospital Medicine (SHM), which focuses on the world of hospitalists.

The SHM has adopted the following official definition of "Hospitalist": Hospitalists are physicians whose primary professional focus is the general medical care of hospitalized patients.

—Statement on the Society of Hospital Medicine web site

Hospitalists take the handoff of a patient from their primary care physician or the emergency medicine physician who admitted the patient to the hospital. And then later they hand off the care back to the primary care physician. But during the hospital stay itself, the hospitalist takes the lead responsibility for a patient's care.

"Clearly our job and our world view is not to get in the way or contravene anything the primary care doctor is doing, but often the hospitalization has its own flavor and tempo. People ask a lot at the beginning, 'Are you carrying out the primary care doctor's orders?' And in many ways the answer is no. In many ways, the hospitalization is a distinct entity," Dr. Wachter says.

At the UCSF Medical Center, Dr. Wachter supervises a team that includes a resident, two interns, two medical students, and a pharmacy student. Their patients are seen also by an army of nurses and physical therapists. And from time to time, patients will be seen by members of a roving band of subspecialists from the worlds of neurology or endocrinology or hematology or radiology or any of the other "-ologies."

Dr. Wachter says hospital patients often have no idea that anyone has any central authority over the crowd of health care professionals that come in and out of their rooms. That job of coordinating everyone and everything is what a hospitalist does. Because hospitalists are a relatively new phenomenon in medical care, Dr. Wachter says he is sometimes hesitant to use the title with new patients.

"When I explain myself to patients when I meet them for the first time, I usually say that 'I'll be your orchestra conductor,'" he says.

He also tells patients that they will get a survey form just before they are discharged, "and one of the first questions is, 'Did you have the sense that anybody was in charge when you were in the hospital?' and I want you to answer yes, because it's me," Dr. Wachter says.

He says the term hospitalist is becoming more familiar to patients. As he was going through his explanation of his role to one patient, the patient's wife piped up, "Oh, so you're a hospitalist."

Hospitalists become intimately familiar with the culture and quirks of their hospital.

"When you are there all day long, you know how the place works. When you can't find the social worker, you know where she

235

goes out for her coffee. The radiologist may owe you a favor. All that informal stuff that you can't explain on an organizational chart, and yet is the way real work gets done," Dr. Wachter says.

Dr. House knows the angles. In "The Mistake" (2-08), he wants a transplant surgeon to take a risky case. However, the surgeon thinks the procedure would be doomed to fail and declines the case. Then Dr. House puts some inside knowledge to use . . . but with a dark spin that Dr. Wachter would certainly not condone: He threatens to tell the surgeon's wife about his affairs with nurses. The surgeon caves in to Dr. House's blackmail.

The best use of the intimate knowledge a hospitalist has of the institution and its staff is to forge strong collaboration, in order to manage the immense complexity of hospital care.

"There is a much, much greater appreciation now than there was in the past that medicine is a team sport; that the days of the macho doctor making proclamations and everybody scurrying around carrying out his or her orders, those days need to die as quickly as possible, because they are not the way health care is provided," Dr. Wachter says.

"We've come to recognize that while some of the patients' outcomes have to do with how brilliant their doctor is, it's probably not the majority. The majority of it is how well the system works and how well people work together. That's a lesson other industries learned a long time ago, and something that medicine has been slower to come to."

## Nurses

The image of nursing takes a beating on *House, M.D.*

"When nurses and others do appear, they are somewhat portrayed as obstructionists to the brilliant doctor, or as mindless bureaucrats getting in the way of his unfettered brilliance. In real life medical care isn't like that at all. No doctor does well who doesn't actually rely on, and practically venerate, the nurses around them; because it doesn't happen without them and the full cast of professionals," says AHRQ Director Dr. Clancy.

Dr. House's attitude is captured in "Spin" (2-06). He gives a patient who can't stand up an injection that momentarily restores normal muscle control. The patient stands, but then as the effect fades, he collapses to the floor. Dr. House just looks at the patient, but doesn't try to help him back to bed.

"This is exactly why I created nurses. Clean up on aisle three!" Dr. House bellows.

If instead of lording over the fictional Princeton-Plainsboro Teaching Hospital, Dr. House were practicing at the University Medical Center at Princeton, he would have to answer to Chief Nursing Officer Joanne Ritter-Teitel, Ph.D., R.N.

"I would have that physician in my office, and there would be a discussion about what appropriate communication is, and how I would not accept that kind of behavior, that all members of the health team bring value to our patients, whether it is a housekeeper or the person who brings the dietary tray or the nurse or the physician," she says.

Dr. House's treatment of nurses doesn't win any fans at the Center for Nursing Advocacy in Baltimore, Maryland.

"That's really a very limited view of nursing and they tend to show only the most unskilled aspects of nursing," says Executive Director Sandy Summers, R.N., M.S.N., M.P.H.

In "Daddy's Boy" (2-05), Foreman is examining a patient.

"What's that smell?" he asks.

When he pulls back the sheets on the bed, he sees that the patient has soiled them.

"We're going to need a nurse," Foreman says.

"Yes, nurses do clean up patients' stool," Summers says. "But you'd never know from watching House that you might actually find signs of a life-threatening illness when you are cleaning up a patient's stool. Maybe they have liver disease or a gall bladder disease or maybe they are having intestinal bleeding or maybe a parasite."

Indeed, the type of parasitic tapeworm that was the cause of the patient's illness in the first episode of *House, M.D.* is frequently spotted by nurses checking patient stools.

In "Three Stories" (1-21), Dr. House is the patient in a flashback to the infarction that crippled his leg. He is in a hospital bed when he feels symptoms of an abnormal heart rhythm. The heart monitor next to the bed is indicating the beginning of a rapid and dangerous heartbeat known as wide complex tachycardia. He tells the nurse to give him an injection, but she hesitates. As monitor alarms sound, he passes out.

Dr. Cuddy rushes into the room and asks the nurse, "What have you got?"

"Wide complex tachycardia."

Dr. Cuddy seems baffled that the nurse would know how to recognize it.

"Who diagnosed it?" she asks.

"He did," the nurse replies, looking at Dr. House.

"What do they mean '*he* did'?" Summers says. "Nurses can read the monitors and they often read them far better than physicians do. Nurses are often in the position of teaching physicians, especially younger ones, what these rhythms are and how to identify them. Nurses see these rhythms day after day after day and can often identify them very quickly."

She also points out that while Dr. House and his fellows are routinely shown giving injections and other treatments to patients, in reality that is not how things usually work.

"Physicians prescribe the medicines, or advanced practice nurses prescribe the medications, and then staff nurses deliver them. It's an essential check and balance; one person prescribes it and a second person, the nurse, is supposed to double-check to make sure the medication is good for the patient, that it is not something that will counteract one of the other medications the patient is getting and won't interact to cause major side effects. And they make sure it goes in the right IV. It can be very complex, when a patient has five different IVs and twenty-five different medications, to figure out which medications are compatible with each other."

Summers points out that nurses are with a patient, or nearby, throughout the hospital stay. They look at the color and texture of the skin, how the patient is breathing, talking, thinking. It is nurses that literally have their fingers on the pulse of their patients.

"Physicians come in, they spend two minutes with the patient, and then they take off. The nurses are there twenty-four hours a day to help the patients understand their conditions, watch them minute by minute to see how they are doing. The House character seems to be in charge of monitoring as well, which is totally unrealistic," Summers says.

Nurses get a better shake in "Skin Deep" (2-13). The patient's heart stops in the middle of the night. When monitor alarms sound, nurses quickly respond. As one confirms the cardiac arrest with a stethoscope, another nurse prepares an injection to revive the patient.

Summers says Dr. House's general attitude toward nurses is not entirely fictional. She says physicians who treat nurses poorly are partly to blame for the nation's nursing shortage, by creating stressful working conditions that lead to burnout.

So how would Summers like working with Dr. House? Her response is surprising.

"I think he would be a breath of fresh air compared to many of the physicians we have to work with," she says. "He does mock his coworkers and says obnoxious things to them, but he is at least witty; and that would be the breath of fresh air. There are way too many physicians who are plenty obnoxious and belittling and imperious, without a shred of wit."

## Leading Hospitals into a New Era

Even as hospitals emphasize teamwork and the value of every member of that team, Dr. Wachter at the UCSF Medical Center says he and other hospitalists have a responsibility to lead a fundamental transformation in how hospitals are structured and managed.

"As a hospitalist, you have two patients. One is the patient. The second is the hospital. Part of what you are here for, part of the way you add value is that you make the system work better for everybody," he says.

When Edward Vogler took over as chairman of the board of Princeton-Plainsboro Teaching Hospital for part of the first season of *House, M.D.*, he declared that he wanted to change the way the hospital was run. The climax of his campaign was a board meeting called in order to oust Dr. House.

"Gregory House is a symbol of everything wrong with the health care industry. Waste. Insubordination. Doctors preening like they're kings and the hospital their own private fiefdom. Health care is a business; I'm gonna run it like one. I hereby move to revoke the tenure of Dr. Gregory House and terminate his employment at this hospital, effective immediately," Vogler declared in "Babies and Bathwater" (1-18).

Vogler failed to get rid of Dr. House, but elements of his tirade against imperious physicians resonate with other reformers. To Dr. Wachter, the character of Dr. House is a dinosaur.

"In some ways, it is a vision from years past of the doctor as the iconoclastic, brilliant, virtuoso free spirit, who does it his own way and the hospital is there to do his bidding. He is a little bit caricaturized, but that is not that far off from the way many doctors in the past were acculturated to expect the system to work. And frankly, on the opposite side, many CEOs went to school to learn how to keep doctors happy."

He says that although *House, M.D.* overdramatizes the situation, the old incentives of the hospital business encouraged that kind of behavior.

"It's almost flabbergasting now when you think about it, but that was the nature of the beast. The hospital was sort of the hobby shop where doctors came in and did their work. And because the doctors brought in the business, the hospital's job was to make sure that the doctors were as happy as they could be, because the docs could take their business elsewhere," Dr. Wachter says.

Dr. Wachter and others say medicine can learn valuable lessons from the history of the aerospace industry.

## From Yeager to Glenn

Shortly after World War II, Chuck Yeager became the first person to fly faster than the speed of sound. Even though he was just part of a huge government project, Yeager still embodied many of the attitudes of the barnstormers of aviation's earliest days. He relied heavily on his individual skill and instincts to stay alive as he pushed the frontiers of flying.

Just days before his historic supersonic flight, Yeager broke some ribs. Rather than play it safe, Yeager kept quiet about his injury to make sure no one replaced him on the record-breaking attempt. Because of his injury, Yeager couldn't use his right arm to close the aircraft hatch. He confided in a coworker, who sawed off a broomstick, so that Yeager could reach the latch with his left arm.

Yeager did break the sound barrier on that day in 1946. But the way he put his interests ahead of those of the program, broke the rules, and deceived his superiors all sound very reminiscent of Dr. House's attitude. In other words, success is the ultimate excuse. That same sort of individual pride also contributed to the deaths of many pilots and passengers in those days.

The first American to orbit the earth was a very different kind of pilot. John Glenn, who went on to become a U.S. senator, did not see individual prowess as the deciding factor between success and failure.

"It was a very different vision of what it meant to be a great pilot: You were a team player," Dr. Wachter says. "Glenn was trained as an engineer. You embraced checklists. You embraced redundancies in the system. You didn't believe that you were flawless; you recognized that you were a member of a team.

"And in many ways medicine is at the cusp of that transformation. There is no doubt in my mind that the great doctor of the future will look much less like House and much more like John Glenn: certainly a leader of a team, but a team player, a collaborator, someone who thinks about systems, someone who doesn't believe they are impervious to errors, but actually recognizes that they are error prone and that the only way to keep things safe is to create a system that anticipates everybody's errors and catches them."

The transformation of aviation was not just about protecting test pilots. It has been part of dramatic improvements in air travel safety. In the 1950s, the rate of fatal air crashes for commercial airliners was around one per 400,000 departures. In other words, on average there would be about 400,000 safe flights between crashes. By the end of the century, the fatal crash rate had dropped to less than one-tenth as much. There are now almost 5 million safe flights for every one that crashes and kills a passenger.

The eyes of the pilots flying planes today are not any sharper. Their reflexes are not any quicker. It's true that aircraft are built better now; but a big reason for the safety improvement is change in the overall system and attitudes about the role of pilots.

Dr. Wachter says he got a sense of the important cultural differences between modern flying and medicine when a group of airline pilots visited the UCSF Medical Center and watched some surgeries. He says the pilots were impressed by the skill of the surgeons and others involved, as well as by the pace of the surgeries and the sophisticated medical technology. But then came some telling questions.

"They asked the nurses, 'How do you set up the operating room for a hip replacement or a cardiac bypass surgery?' or 'What's the process for getting informed consent?' And what the nurses said was, 'Oh, for Dr. Smith we do it this way. For Dr. Jones, he likes us to do it that way.' And the pilots were flabbergasted, because they said that would be inconceivable in aviation, to walk into a cockpit of a 747 and say, 'I want it set up this particular way, because I like it better that way.' They have recognized how fundamentally chaotic and unsafe that is."

Today's airline pilots are willing to give up some individual freedom and authority, and accept standards and uniformity, in order to reduce the number of potentially fatal errors.

"That of course would be foreign to House and antithetical to everything he stands for. But the way we are increasingly trying to train physicians is exactly the opposite of his world view," Dr. Wachter says.

Foreman says, "House! You can't do this!"

"Oh, if I had a nickel for every time I've heard that," Dr. House replies.

—"Distractions" (2-12)

Barnstorming fighter pilots who break all the rules and yet live to fight another day are certainly far more exciting than jumbo-jet captains.

And so a brilliant medical renegade like Dr. House, who smashes through bureaucracy and medical convention in his individual battle to save his patients, is far more interesting than methodical physicians who check the latest guidelines and protocols, while trying not to do more harm than good with their tests and treatments.

But when you board a plane to cross the country, do you want excitement or an uneventful flight that gets you safe and sound to the destination listed on your ticket? And if you ever have to check into a hospital, with your life in the balance, which kind of physician do you really want controlling your care?

# EPILOGUE

*House, M.D.* is a television show, a piece of entertaining drama and comedy. Yet even though it is fiction, the stories embody our hopes and our fears about health and sickness, conflict and rescue. The plots play off our knowledge and beliefs of the world . . . in this case, the world of medicine.

After reading this overview of some of the aspects of medicine portrayed in the show, I hope you have a bit more knowledge of modern medicine and a bit more understanding of the distinctions between the kernels of truth and the flights of exaggeration the characters dramatize, so that you can savor an informed taste of the cocktail of reality and fantasy that play out in each story of *House, M.D.*

# INDEX

Abdominal pain, 14
"Acceptance," 146, 171, 177
Acetaminophen, brand names for, 203
Addiction
    behaviors of, 211
    dosage and, 204
    fear of, 205–6
    high risk conditions for, 211
    of House, 207
    physician training in, 207
    of physicians, 207–8
    population disorders of, 205
    undertreatment and, 205
    warning signs of, 209–10, 211
*Advances in Skin & Wound Care*, 152
Albendazole, 117
Alcohol
    course for controlling, 207
    physician abuse of, 206–11
Alkaptonuria, 122
Allitt, Beverly, 12
AMA. *See* American Medical Association
Ambulance, 20–22
    Advanced Life Support for, 162
    heart attack treatment in, 20–21
American Medical Association (AMA), 103,
    158, 177–78, 182, 186, 205
ANA (antinuclear antibody test), 104
Andrews, Billy, 43
Anemia, 112, 154. *See also* Aplastic anemia
Aneurysm, 35, 202
Angiostatin, 134–35
Angood, Peter, 230–31
Anthrax attacks, 49
Antiangiogenesis drugs, 135
Antibiotics, 113–14, 117, 140, 177
Anticonvulsant drugs, 185
Antiviral drugs, 185
Aphasia, 9
Aplastic anemia, 93
Applegate, W.B., 58
Arsenic, 94

Arthritis, 164
Aspirin, 143
Asthma, 35
Ativan, 6–8
Auscultation, 43, 99
Automatic external defibrillators (AEDs),
    21–22, 162
"Autopsy," 111
Aviation, 242–43

"Babies and Bathwater," 16, 32, 135, 161,
    190, 195, 240
Baer, William, 152
Barnea, Eytan R., 193
Benzodiazepines, seizures and, 209
Bevacizumab, 135
Biomedical research, 167–68
Biopsies, 66–70, 118, 155
    of lungs, 69–70
    needle, 110, 111
    retinal, 66
    stereotactic needle, 69
BioSense, 49
Birth control pills, 147
Blood, 66
Blood pressure, 30
BMP (basic metabolic panel). *See* CHEM-7
Bomback, Andrew, 37
Bone diseases
    from cadmium, 140–42
    Fanconi's syndrome, 141
    osteomyelitis, 152
Borgstede, James, 77–78, 79
Bowel disease, 37–38
Braddock, Clarence H., 189
Brandt, Lawrence J., 218, 220
Brant-Zawadzki, Michael, 79
BRCA1 test, 56–57, 64
Breathing, difficulty, 17
Bronchitis, 35
Bronchoscope, 69–70
Bulimia nervosa, 127–29

# INDEX

Cadmium, 140–42
  in cigarettes, 142
  legal levels of, 141–42
  in marijuana/hemp, 142
Cameron, 34–35, 49, 59, 65, 79, 88, 93, 94,
  103, 120, 139, 157, 171, 178, 189,
  195–96, 233
Campbell, Craig, 184–85
Cancer(s), 2, 13, 33, 61, 71–72, 74, 79, 83,
  105, 115, 118, 146
  5-year survival rate of, 163–64
  blood, 119, 132
  breast, 38, 56–57, 64, 81, 89, 97, 122,
    148, 149–50, 155, 159, 164, 192–93
  cervical, 60, 193–94
  early detection of, 164
  interspecies differences in, 135
  lead-time bias in, 34, 164
  leukemia, 61
  lung, 33–34, 38–39, 72, 79, 89–90, 122,
    135, 161, 163, 171, 190–92
  pregnancy and, 190–94
  prostate, 69, 97, 110, 111, 163, 164, 182
  skin, 163
  symptoms of, 39–40
*Cancer and Pregnancy* (Barnea), 193
Caplan, Arthur, 179, 180–81
Carbamazepine, 68
Cardiologists, 150, 202
Cardiomyopathy, 128
Case-based reasoning, 92
CAT (computed axial tomography). *See* CT
  (computed tomography)
Cataracts, sunflower, 109
CBC (complete blood count), 61–62
CDC. *See* U.S. Centers for Disease Control
  and Prevention
*Cecil Textbook of Medicine*, 128
Cerebral malaria, 10
Chandra, Amitabh, 173
Chase, 35, 40, 49, 57, 59, 63, 79, 88, 93,
  109, 117, 133–34, 157, 160, 189, 222,
  233
CHEM-7, 61
Chest pain, 14
Child abuse, reporting, 195–96
Chloramphenicol, 93–94
Cholesterol levels, 58, 164
Chorioretinitis, 67
Chronic disease, 164
Cigarettes
  cadmium in, 142
  cancer and, 163
  heart disease and, 162

  stigma of, 38–39
  for ulcerative colitis/Crohn's disease,
    37–38
Clancy, Carolyn M., 155–57, 232–33, 237
Clinical practice directory, website for, 97
Clinical trial registry, 199–200
Clonazepam, 15
Coiera, Enrico, 86, 89, 90, 91, 92, 97
Communication training, "patient-
  centered," 172
Computers
  assisting physicians, 86–89
  medical applications of, 90–92, 97–98
  medical errors from, 158–59
  systems available, 95–97
Congestive heart failure, 162–63
Consciousness, loss of, 17–18
"Control," 126–27, 129–30, 157, 161, 194,
  199, 218
Cough, 13, 17
*Crossing the Quality Chasm: A New Health
  System for the 21st Century*, 160
Cryptosporidium, 46
CT (computed tomography), 71–72, 74, 83,
  89, 111, 116, 118, 166
  cost of, 77
  health care plans and, 78–79
  overuse of, 76–79
Cuddy, Lisa, 24, 55, 169–70, 173, 178–79,
  195, 199, 212, 214, 218, 238
  timid behavior of, 209, 210, 216,
    223–24
  unlikely behavior of, 227
Culliton, Barbara, 167
"Cursed," 139, 179
Cushing's disease, 161
Cystic fibrosis, 11, 64

"Daddy's Boy," 63, 103, 120, 123, 126,
  157, 161, 171, 237
"Damned If You Do," 37, 156, 188
*Dartmouth Atlas of Health Care*, 148–51
"Deception," 11
"Decision Theory for Clinicians: Uses and
  Misuses of Clinical Tests" (Applegate),
  58
Dengue fever, 2
Depression, 2, 13, 112
"Detox," 189, 209
Diabetes, 112, 151, 164, 203
Diagnosis, vii-viii, 1–3, 42–43, 86, 102–3,
  106–7, 117, 202–3
  clinicians v. academics, 106
  by computer, 91–92, 94, 95–97, 97

differential, 2, 101–3, 104, 105–6, 112, 115, 120, 125
emergency, 16–17
heuristics and, 121–25
hurrying, 121
occupation and, 123–24
Osler teaching, 43–44
process of, 4–6, 8–10, 12
six steps of, 102–3
subtle clues for, 119–20
technological tools for, ix, 100
undifferentiated problem and, 3–4
Diagnosticians, 234
"Distractions," 152, 223, 243
Dizziness, 13, 118
"DNR," 114–15, 180
Doppler effect, 75
Double blind design, 146
Drugs, 127, 144
animal tests for, 134–35, 138
benefits v. side effects of, 136–37
bioavailabilities of, 134
cost of, 167
course for controlling, 206–7
dosage of, 134, 204, 209
emergency use of, 137–38
experimental, 133–39, 138
human clinical trials for, 136–37
laboratory testing of, 133–34
mix-ups in, 157
multiple research studies on, 199–200
opioid, 203–4, 205
overuse of, 150
for pain, 203–6
patches/pumps for, 205
physician abuse of, 206–11
withdrawal symptoms of, 209
Dubay, Inga, 158
DXplain, 96
*Dying for a Drink: What You and Your Family Should Know About Alcoholism* (Spickard), 207

Edelstein, Ludwig, 175
Eflornithine, 94
Eisenberg, John, 232–33
Electrocardiograms, 91
Emergency room, 16–19
ambulances as, 20–22
presenting problems in, 17–20
in U.S., 19–20
Emetine, 128
Encainide, 144
Endostatin, 134–35

Epidemic Intelligence Service (EIS), 45–47, 51–52
Epilepsy, 6–8
Epinephrine, 156
"Evidence-based medicine," 143–48
agency providing, 154–56
case reports/series and, 145
confounding factor in, 145
expert opinion and, 144
observational studies, 145
randomized controlled trials and, 145–46
systematic reviews for, 147–48

Factitious illnesses. *See* Munchausen syndrome
"Failure to Communicate," 9, 94–95, 228–29
Fallowfield, Lesley, 172
Fatigue, 13
Federal Drug Administration (FDA), 84
Fen-phen diet drug, 136–37
Fever, 17, 18, 22–23
FUO (of unknown origin), 118–19
"Fidelity," 1, 36, 92, 93, 145
Fishman, Elliot, 75–76, 78, 79
Flecainide, 144
Flu, 2, 102
swine, vaccination, 104–5
Fomepizole, for ethylene glycol poisoning, 147
Forearm fractures, 149
Foreman, 49, 59, 66, 79, 88, 93, 94, 104, 120, 133, 137, 157, 173, 177, 178, 183–84, 185, 200, 222, 233
Frist, Bill, 19

Gascon, Generosa G., 68
Genetic tests, 63–65
Getty, Barbara, 158
GIDEON (Global Infectious Diseases and Epidemiology Network), 95–96
Gilbert, David N., 105, 117, 233
Glenn, John, as team player, 242
Glucose, 61, 74
Goldman, Lee, 234
*Guide to Health Informatics* (Coiera), 89
Guillain-Barré syndrome, 104–5, 112–13

Hantavirus, 47–48
*Harrison's Principles of Internal Medicine, 16th edition*, 107, 170
Headaches, 42–43, 110

Health, 132
  literacy, 186–87
  major transition of, 164
  survival and, 129–30
Health care
  acute/chronic conditions and, 164
  cost increases of, 166–67, 173
  curative paradigm of, 167
  end of life variations of, 187
  ethics and, 180
  expectations of, 213
  flexibility of, 155–56
  heart disease prevention by, 162–63
  high-tech medical model of, 168
  impaired physicians in, 210
  insurance, 213
  oaths for, 173–77
  overuse of, 150–51
  personnel required for, 167
  place of death variations in, 187–88
  preemptive medicine for, 167–68
  scientific evidence and, 151, 155–57
  tactics v. values in, 187
  teamwork of, 181, 233
  in U.S., 19, 168
*Health Care USA: Understanding Its Organization and Delivery* (Sultz, Young), 212–13
Heart attack, 14, 17, 102, 110–11, 146, 150, 151, 164, 181
  ambulance treatment for, 20–21
  angioplasty/cardiac stents for, 73
  death rates of, 161–63
  disease underlying, 162–63
  online risk assessment for, 98
  prescriptions for, 149
  prevention of, 162
  from Vioxx, 199
  as zebra, 26
Heart transplants, 127, 128, 161
  availability of, 130–32
  "extended criteria" for, 132
  infection and, 130–32
  survival rates of, 129–30
"Heavy," 21, 161
Hemp, environmental use of, 142
Hepatitis A, 49
Hepatitis B, 131–32
Hepatitis C, 130–32, 133
Heroin, 204
Heuristics
  anchoring/adjustments, 124–25
  availability, 121–22
  "cognitive illusions" and, 121–26
  looking for confirmation, 125

  as practical, 120–21
  representativeness, 123–24
Hickson, Gerald, 172–73
Hillman, Bruce, 78–79
Hip fractures, 148–49
Hippocrates, 173, 218
Hippocratic Oath (classical), 173–75
*The Hippocratic Oath: Text, Translation, and Interpretation* (Edelstein), 175
Hirudin, danger of, 154
"Histories," 156, 179, 215
HIV/AIDS, 2, 11, 13, 104, 132, 133, 139, 159, 161
Holmes, Sherlock, vii
Hospitalists, 233–36, 240
Hospitals
  authorities for, 228–29
  building boom of, 213
  decision enforcement at, 221
  dress code of, 218–21
  enforcement actions against, 228
  expense/sophistication of, 213
  governance process in, 222–23
  history of, 213
  inspections of, 228
  Joint Commission reviews of, 230–32
  licenses for, 227
  medical teams in, 235, 240
  microbes in, 113–14
  ownership of, 213–14
  parallel hierarchy of, 217
  physician reporting at, 221
  services in, 214
  standards/uniformity in, 243
  technology in, 213
  transformation of, 240–41, 242
  unlike businesses, 212, 216
House, Gregory, vii-viii, 1–4, 8–10, 14, 16, 23, 25–27, 32, 34–35, 37–38, 44–45, 49, 65, 67, 75, 79, 88, 91–94, 102, 106, 123, 129–32, 135, 139–40, 145–47, 152, 155, 157, 161, 171, 228–29
  administrator relationships of, 216
  antibiotic prescriptions of, 113
  blackmail by, 236
  computer replacing, 86
  crises of, 161
  diagnosis by, 126–27
  dishonesty of, 189, 194–95
  evaluations of, 179–81
  evidence-based medicine and, 144
  as exciting/dangerous, 243–44
  infarction of, 201–3, 238
  law violations by, 195–96

medication of, 203, 204
nurses and, 237–40
as old-fashioned, 240–41, 243
"outrageous" behavior of, 223–25
pain of, 203
patience of, 115
patient talks with, 30
preferences of, 150
as problem, 206–7, 230–31
rules ignored by, 221
skill/behavior of, 169–70, 173, 177,
   178–79, 188–89
students disdained by, 214–15
test/treatment threshold of, 111–12, 114–15
*House, M.D.*, viii, 1, 8–10, 17, 27, 44–48,
   53–54, 58–60, 62–63, 66, 83, 116, 120,
   122, 153, 157, 181, 185, 200, 221, 233
bizarre cases on, 102, 132, 155, 156, 202
clinic scenes on, 28
"diagnosis room" on, 101
nursing image on, 236–37
patients on, 127
realism of, 76, 79
time warp on, 65
treatment on, 112–13, 140, 143
Human clinical trials
phases of, 136–37
Thalidomide shortcuts in, 138–40
volunteers/website for, 138
Human experimentation, 199
"Humpty Dumpty," 23–24
"Hunting," 65, 161, 178
Huntington's Disease, 64–65, 107
Hydatid disease, 80
Hydrocodone, brand names for, 203
Hypothyroidism, 112

Identification of the Impaired Physician, 211
Imaging, 91, 118
clinical directory for, 97
computers analyzing, 89–90
cost of, 77
CT (computed tomography), 71–72, 74
health care plans and, 77–79
MRI (magnetic resonance imaging),
   70–71, 75
nuclear medicine scans, 73–75
overuse of, 76–79
ultrasound, 75–80
Immunosuppressive drugs, side effects of, 127
Infarction. *See also* Heart attack
myocardial, 202
of skeletal muscles, 202–3
treatment for, 202

Infectious diseases, ix, 6, 17, 46–51, 140
antibiotics for, 113–14
cerebral malaria as, 10
children and, 165
HIV, 2, 11, 13, 104, 132–33, 139, 159,
   161
technology and, 47, 48–49
tracking outbreaks of, 45–49
transplants and, 130–32
Informed consent, 182–89
ample time for, 185
communication for, 183–87
forms for, 186–87
law of, 182
weak literacy/language skills and, 186
Injuries, 6–7, 17
Interferon, 68
International Classification of Sleep Disorders, 15
Intrauterine device (IUD), 5
Intraventricular interferon, 183–86
alternatives to, 185–86
risks/complications of, 185
Ipecac, syrup of, 127–29, 194
abuse of, 127–29
research on, 129
Italic handwriting, 158

Jaundice, 14
Jenkins, Valerie, 172
Joint Commission on Accreditation of
   Healthcare Organization (JCAHO), 31,
   229–32
*Journal of the American Medical
   Association*, 172–73, 186, 189, 198, 201
"Judgment under Uncertainty: Heuristics and
   Biases" (Tversky, Kahneman), 121

Kahneman, Daniel, 121, 124
Kellerman, Rick, 3, 5, 8–9, 29, 31, 44, 112,
   115
Kelly, James, 9–10
Kelsey, Frances, 138, 139–40
Kveim-Siltzbach test, 65

Lab coat, white, 224
hypertension and, 219
microbes on, 220
practicality of, 218
for students, 219–20
as symbol, 218
Laboratory tests, 54–59, 106–7, 125
common, 60–85
computer directory for, 97

Laboratory tests (*cont.*)
by computers, 89
expertise for, 59–60
false positive/negative, 77–78, 80–83, 104, 110
misleading, 58–59
overuse of, 150
PSA, 110, 111, 164
selection process for, 55–56, 62
sensitivity/specificity of, 80–83
special animals for, 135–36
thresholds, 109–10
Laënnec, René Théophile Hyacinthe, 41
Lambert-Eaton myasthenic syndrome, 32
*The Lancet*, 93
Leeches, 152–54
anemia from, 154
clotting prevention by, 153–54
*as hirudo medicinalis*, 153
for reconstructive surgery, 154
risks of, 154
in wild, 154
Legionella pneumophila, 46
Leprosy (Hansen's disease), 139
Lhermitte's sign, 120
Lidocaine injections, for hearts, 143–44
Life expectancy, 165–66
childhood deaths and, 165
health care and, 165–66
living conditions and, 165
senior years and, 166
in U.S., 168
Liver disease, 108–9
Lorazepam, 7
"Love Hurts," 35
Lumpectomy, 148
Lupus, 104
Lyme disease, 104

Maggots, 152–54
blow flies for, 152–53
for debridement, 152
dosage of, 152
secretions of, 152
Malaria, 10, 90, 94–95
Malingering, 11
Malpractice premiums, 173
Mammograms, 81, 89, 155, 164
*Manual of Family Practice* (Taylor), 31
Marijuana *(cannabis sativa)*
cadmium in, 142
environmental use of, 142
Markel, Howard, 99–100, 175

Mastectomies, 148. *See also* Cancers
"Maternity," 133, 221
Measles, 132, 185
mutant, 66–68
Medicaid, complexity of, 229
Medical education, 43–44
authorities for, 229
critical thinking for, 121
Medical errors, 156–61
from computers, 158–59
in drug prescriptions, 157
from handwriting, 157–59
in operations, 157
research on, 159–61
routine, 156–57
solutions for, 160–61
"Medical Professionalism in the New Millennium: A Physician Charter," 176–77
Medical records
electronic, 91
probability networks for, 91
in U.S., 19–20
Medical research
bad results burying, 199–200
changes in, 167–68
increasing articles on, 87
industry funding and, 197–200
marketing spin in, 199
Medical search engines, 86–87, 93. *See also* Medline
Medicare, 230
Medline, 86–87
Melarsoprol, 94
Meningococcal meningitis, 17
Meperidine, 208
*Merck Manual*, 87–88
Methanol poisoning, 146–47
Miller Fisher syndrome, 104–5
"The Mistake," 160, 222, 236
"Mob Rules," 34, 133–34, 170
Mononucleosis, 112
Morphine, 203
sustained-release, 204–5
MRI (magnetic resonance imaging), 70–71, 75, 89, 110, 111, 116, 155, 166, 177, 202
cost of, 83
implants and, 84
metal and, 83–84
overuse of, 76–79, 150
safety of, 83–85
Muller, Carolyn, 194
Multilingual U.S., 23–24
Multiple sclerosis, 2, 103–4, 105, 120

Munchausen syndrome, 11–12
Münchhausen, Karl Friedrich von, 10–11
Myoclonic jerk, 67–68, 88, 185

Narcotics Anonymous, Twelve Steps of, 207
National Institutes of Health (NIH)
    knowledge/technology of, 166–67
    outside payment policy of, 197
Neural networks, 90–91
Neurocysticercosis, 116–17
Neurologists, 1, 44, 184
*Neurology and General Medicine*, 10
Neuropathies, 2
Neurosurgeons, 173, 185
*New England Journal of Medicine*, 37, 99,
    131, 175, 186, 199, 234
Nocturnal eating/drinking (Dagwood) syn-
    drome, 15
Non-Hodgkin's lymphoma, 119
Normal, meaning of, 57–58
Norwalk virus, 124
Nowack, William J., 6–8
Nuclear medicine scans, 70, 73–75, 117
    PET (positron-emission tomography),
        74–75, 83, 89
    SPECT (single photon emission com-
        puted tomography), 74–75
Nurses
    pilots questioning, 243
    real life physicians and, 239–40
    skills of, 238–39
    valuing, 237

Oaascge-Orlow, Michael K., 186
Obesity, 153
O'Brien, Richard, 16–18, 21
Obstetricians, 173
Occam's razor, 121
Office visits
    chief complaints during, 28–30
    top-to-bottom exam during, 30–32
Olfactory neuroepithelium, 142
Omega-3 fatty acids, 155
Ommaya reservoir, 183–86
    risks of, 184
    surgical procedure of, 183
Oncologist, ix, 80
Ophthalmologist, 67
Opium, 204
Oral isoprinosine (inosiplex), 68
Organ donation
    best practices of, 225–27
    family veto power for, 226
Osler, William, 42, 43–44

Osteomyelitis, 152
Osteoporosis, 73

Pain
    abdominal, 14, 17
    back, 14
    chest, 17, 21, 73, 102, 107, 110–11
    chest, emergent, 13–14
    drug withdrawal and, 209
    drugs for, 203–6
    medication abuse, 205–11
    opioid drugs for, 203–4
    pelvic region, 14
    undertreatment of, 205
    Vioxx for, 137, 199
    as vital sign, 31
Pap smear tests, 60, 194
Papillomaviruses, 194
Paraneoplastic syndromes, 32–34, 105, 190
Parasomnias, 14–15
Parkinson's disease, 107
"Paternity," 4, 55, 65, 66–68, 88, 183, 185
Pathologists, 60, 167
Patients
    after crisis outcomes of, 161–64, 162–63
    clinical drug trials for, 138
    daily life survey of, 5
    death from errors, 159–60
    decision support websites for, 97–98
    decision-making by, 189
    directives of, 180–82
    early detection and, 164
    end of life desires of, 187–88
    excessive health care for, 150
    handwashing requests by, 221
    information for, 182
    informed consent of, 182–89
    occupation of, 123–24
    physician attire and, 220
    physician encounter with, 4–6
    physician trust by, 170–71
    physician's communication with, 22–25,
        181–82
    physician's handwriting and, 157–59
    physicians interrupting, 4–5, 40–41
    physician's relationship with, 8–10, 16
    preferences of, 150
    website credibility for, 98
PDA (personal data assistants), 87–89
Pharmaceutical companies
    marketing campaigns of, 200–201
    physician support by, 197–201
    promotional spending of, 201
Phlebotomists, 66

Physical exams, 106–7
    abdomen, 36
    breast, 36
    chest, 35
    doorknob questions in, 40–41
    duration/rhythm of, 39
    ear, 34
    environmental, 45
    eye, 32, 116, 139
    heart, 35
    on *House, M.D.*, 45
    legs, 36
    lymph nodes, 35
    mouth, 34
    neck, 34–35
    neurological, 36–37
    pelvic/hernia/genital/rectal/prostate, 37
    physician preparation for, 41
    smell check during, 37
    symptoms in, 39–40
    technology influencing, 41–42, 52–53
"Physician Charter," 176–77
Physicians, viii-ix, 233–36, 240
    addictions of, 207–8
    amenable to change, 156
    attire of, 218–21
    bad news communication by, 171–72
    capital punishment facilitated by, 177–78
    communication skills of, 170–72
    communication training for, 171–72
    complaints unresolved by, 44
    computer assisted, 86–88, 88–89, 92
    counseling/courses for, 223
    death and, 171
    emergency, ix, 1, 16–19, 102, 107–8, 234
    family, ix, 4–5, 44
    freedom/authority of, 242–43
    goal of, 125
    handwashing by, 221
    handwriting of, 157–59
    home treatment by, 213
    hospital privileges and, 217
    hurrying, 121
    impaired, 203–11, 210
    information overload for, 85, 87–88, 92
    informed consent and, 182–87
    interruptions by, 4–5, 40–41
    licenses for, 228
    malpractice lawsuits for, 172–73
    medical errors of, 159–61
    as non employees, 217
    oaths for, 173–77
    patient communication with, 22–25
    patient decision-making and, 189
    patient encounter with, 4–6
    patient trust for, 170–71
    patient's occupation and, 123–24
    patient's relationship with, 8–10
    patient's values honored by, 188
    peer/admin reviews of, 222–23
    pharmaceutical spending on, 201
    physical exam preparation for, 41
    physician for, 207–8
    preferences of, 150
    prescribing opioids, 205
    primary care, 2–3, 13–14, 44, 234
    reporting abuse by, 208
    as sales force, 217
    specialists, ix, 1–2, 44, 97, 167
    substance abuse by, 205–11
    unwarranted variations by, 147–51
PKU (phenylketonuria), 64
Plague, 95–96
Plasmapheresis, 112–13
Pneumonia, 35, 90, 179
Poison, 127–29, 140
    methanol, 146–47
"Poison," 47, 63, 137, 173, 189
Presentation, 2–3, 4
    emergency, problems, 17
    primary care, problems, 12–14
Princeton-Plainsboro Teaching Hospital, 214–15
    accreditation review of, 230
    authorities for, 227–28, 229
*Principles and Practice of Medicine* (Osler), 43–44
Probability networks, 91
*Promoting Pain Relief and Preventing Abuse of Pain Medications: A Critical Balancing Act*, 205–6
Protti, Denis J., 88
Psychogenic events (Phantoms), 51–52
Public health laws, 50–51
Pulmonary disease, 151
Pulmonologist, ix
Pulse, 30

Rabies, 132
Radiation therapy, 120, 148
    for pregnant women, 191–93
Radiologists, 2, 79, 81, 89–90, 167
Rales, 35
Reconstructive surgery, 154
Reportable diseases, 47, 49–50
Respiration, 30
Reticulum cell sarcoma, 122
Review of systems, questions for, 29–30

Reye's syndrome, 143
Rhonchi, 35
Ribavirin, 68
Ritter-Teitel, Joanne, 188–89, 223, 237
Rodriguez, Fred H., Jr., 54–55, 56, 59, 60
Roentgen, Wilhelm Conrad, 72
"Role Model," 14, 197
Roosevelt, Franklin D., 27
Rosen, Max, 77
Ruckdeschel, John C., 190–92
Rule-based systems, 90
Rx for Handwriting Success, 158

*The Sanford Guide to Antimicrobial Therapy* (Gilbert), 105
Sarcoidosis, 65
Savage, Seddon R., 203–5
Schizophrenia, 108
Schwarzenegger, Arnold, 179
Scientific evidence
    for antiarrhythmia drugs, 144
    for lidocaine, 143–44
    medical practice and, 143
Scleroderma, 104
"Sed" rate (erythrocyte sedimentation rate, ESR), 60–61, 76
Seizures, 6–8, 116–17
    acute symptomatic, 6
    benzodiazepines and, 209
"Sex Kills," 130–31, 221, 224, 227
Sexsomnia, 14–16
Shapiro, Colin, 15
Sickle-cell anemia, 203
Signs, 30, 125, 170
Sjögren's syndrome, 104
"Skin Deep," 195–96, 239
Sleep
    disorders of, 14–16, 93–94
"Sleeping Dogs Lie," 29
Smith, Harriet, 194
Smoking. *See* Cigarettes
"The Socratic Method," 59, 108–9, 195, 221
Sotos, John, 26–27, 105–6, 119, 122
Sphincter paralysis, 104
Spickard, Anderson, Jr., 206–10
"Spin," 57, 58–59, 237
Splenomegaly, 122
"Sports Medicine," 3, 140, 200
Stacy, 179, 228–29
*Staphylococcus aureus* infections, 113–14
Status epilepticus, 7–8
Steroid treatment, 147
Stethoscopes, 41, 75
    electronic, 98–100

history of, 99–100
    as symbols, 218
    technology replacing, 41
Streptomycin, 93–94
Stress, 5
Strokes, 6
The Student Handbook for the Carolinas
    College of Health Sciences, 219–20
Subacute sclerosing panencephalitis (SSPE), 67–68
    alternatives for, 185–86
    treatment for, 183–86
Substance abuse, by physicians, 206–11
Sultz, Harry, 213
Summer, Sandy, 237–40
Survival rates, 129–30
    5-year, 163–64
    disease-free, 163–64
    overall, 163
    progression-free, 164
Swelling, 14
Symptoms, 2, 30, 102, 112, 117–18, 120, 125, 170
    emergency, 17–18
    Kayser-Fleischer rings, 108
    neurological, 32–33
    in physical exams, 39–40

*Taenia solium*, 116
Takayasu's Arteritis, 76
Tapeworms, viii. *See also* Neurocysticercosis
Taylor, Robert B., 31–32, 34, 39–40, 41, 42
"TB or Not TB," 140
Temperature, 30
Thalidomide, 138–40
    for leprosy (Hansen's disease), 139
    pregnant women and, 137–40
"The Mistake," 40
"Three Stories," 35, 179, 202, 214, 238
3M Sound Analysis Software, 99
Thyroid dysfunction, 35
"Tincture of time," 115, 117–18
*To Err Is Human: Building a Safer Health System*, 159–60
"Tox" (toxicology) screen, 62–63, 128
Toxic exposures, 2
Traub, Bruce, 216–17, 221
Treatment, 107
    angioplasty, 162
    benefits/risks of, 182
    for childhood cancers, 163
    experimental, 133–40
    for infarction, 202

Treatment (*cont.*)
  overuse of, 150
  of pain, 204–6
  of polio vaccine, 165
  for progression-free survival, 164
  scientific, 155–57
  selection of, 132
  for SSPE, 183–86
  steroid, 147
  thresholds, 109–11, 114–15, 125
  uncertainty of, 143
  white coat hypertension and, 219
Trotter, Wilfred Batten Lewis, 119
Trypanosome parasites, 93
Tuberculosis, 50–51, 72, 95
Tularemia ("rabbit fever"), 93–94. *See also*
  Sleep
Tumors, ix, 6, 73–74, 118, 140, 145
  in animals, 135–36
  brain, 26–27, 109–10
  drugs for, 134–35
  early detection of, 164
  hepatic, 80
  lung, 32–33
  prostate, 110–11
  type 2 neurofibromatosis, 63
Tversky, Amos, 121, 124
Tylenol, 203

Ultrasound, 70, 75–80, 77, 99, 118
*Unequal Treatment*, 24–25
University Medical Center at Princeton, 223
  authorities for, 227–28
  management dynamics of, 216–17
  as model, 216–17
  parallel hierarchy of, 217
  physician as vice-president at, 221–22
Unwarranted variations, 148–51
  agency to reduce, 154–56
  effective care underuse in, 149
  in local culture/habits, 148–49
  preference-sensitive care misuse in,
    149–50
  supply-sensitive care overuse in, 150–51
UpToDate, 96–97
U.S. Centers for Disease Control and Prevention (CDC), 45, 47, 49, 113, 186,
  189
U.S. Food and Drug Administration,
  128–29, 136–38, 139–40, 158
  emergency drug use and, 137–38
  regulating maggots/leeches, 152–53

*Users' Guides to the Medical Literature*
  (AMA), 103

VanAmringe, Margaret, 232
Vascular disease, 118
Vasculitis, 76
Vassilyadi, Michael, 185
Ventricular tachycardia rhythm, 18
Vicodin, 86, 203, 209
  alternatives to, 204–5
  risks/benefits of, 205
  sudden withdrawal of, 209
  variable blood levels and, 204
Vioxx pain medication, 137
  misleading research on, 199
viruses, viii
Vitamin deficiency, 2
Vogler, Edward, 169–70, 202, 212
  authority of, 216, 217, 218
  House fired by, 240
  interest conflicts of, 197, 200
  recruiting patients, 199

Wachter, Robert, 233–36, 240–41,
  242–43
Warfarin, 59
Weber, F. Parkes, 102
Wegener's granulomatosis, 117–18
Weight loss, 13
Welby, Marcus, 179–80, 233
Williams, Andy, 196
Wilson, 38, 103, 157, 171, 190
Wilson's disease, 108–9
Woodward, Theodore E., 27

X-ray, 72–73, 74, 75, 83, 117
  angiography, 72–73
  bone density, 73
  CTs v., 73
  mammography, 73

Yale Physician's Oath, 175–76
Yeager, Chuck, individual pride of,
  241–42
*Yersinia pestis* bacterium, 96
Young, Kristina, 213

*Zebra Cards* (Sotos), 26–27, 105, 119
"Zebras," vii, 25–27, 102
Zerhouni, Elias, 167–68